THE SECRET OF CANCER & AIDS

Immunological tolerance in the lymph system

The theory is that the immune system recognizes cancer and HIV as harmless self antigens. This theory seems to have opened up some surprising new options for treatment, discussed at length in this book for both the general public and those in the medical field as well.

Contains helpful information you can use at home. New treatment with new results, for you.

JASON MC KENNA

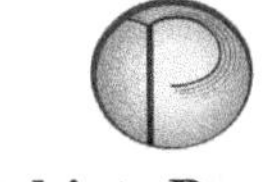

Outskirts Press, Inc.
Denver, Colorado

The opinions expressed in this manuscript are solely the opinions of the author and do not represent the opinions or thoughts of the publisher. The author has represented and warranted full ownership and/or legal right to publish all the materials in this book.

The information in this book is not intended to be used to diagnose or cure any medical condition including cancer, AIDs and HIV without first consulting your healthcare provider. In some cases it may be unwise or detrimental to one's health to boost the immune system if the patient needs to be on, or is on, an immune depressing medication. Always first consult with your medical provider or physician before implementing any options listed in this book. The author and publisher are not responsible for any medical conditions or problems resulting from self treatment or adding to your current treatment plan derived from the information gained in this publication. It is the full responsibility of the reader to first seek and follow the advice given you from your medical provider or physician. This author owns the copywrite and does not permit the reproduction of whole or in part in any form without first obtaining the sole permission of the author.

The Secret of Cancer & AIDS
Immunological tolerance in the lymph system

v2.0

Outskirts Press, Inc.
http://www.outskirtspress.com

ISBN: 978-1-4327-3977-5

PRINTED IN THE UNITED STATES OF AMERICA

Introduction

The first part of this book is about a theory which explains the secret of cancer and AIDS seemingly impregnable immunological invincibility. Once we understand how this happens we can develop a treatment. This book was written as this theory was being developed. Later these developments led to some exciting new options for treatment so these are discussed later.

Reading about these new options for treatment would be useless without knowing how they work, so in order to understand them you would have to read about the theory first.

This theory is so up to date that both it and this book were being developed and written as new information on something called suppressor T cells, was still coming to light. This new information was actually very important in the development of this theory.

Because this book was written as this theory was being

developed and in the order of the research that was done you can follow along and it's like you're right there being completely informed on the situation as it's happening.

Contents

CHAPTER 1

The Theory

Slow Viruses

HIV belongs to a subgroup of retroviruses known as lenti-viruses, or "slow" viruses characterized by a long interval between initial infection and the onset of serious symptoms. Typically, slow viral infections are fatal.

A number of slow virus infections have in fact been caused by conventional viruses. For example, several years after causing measles, the measles virus can be responsible for a rare form of encephalitis called subacute sclerosing panencephalitis (SSPE). One out of every million cases of measles turns into a slow viral infection.

Early Events in HIV Infection

Once HIV enters the body, it infects a large number of CD4+ cells and replicates rapidly. During this acute or primary phase of infection, the blood contains many viral particles that spread throughout the body, seeding various organs, particularly the **lymphoid organs.**

Two to 4 weeks after exposure to the virus, up to 70 percent of HIV-infected people suffer flu-like symptoms related to the acute infection. Their immune system fights back with **killer T cells (CD8+ T cell**s) and **antibodies**, which dramatically reduce HIV levels. According to this information, the immune system could easily win if only it continued to attack the virus as it did to begin with. A person's CD4+ T cell count may rebound somewhat and even approach its original level. A person may then remain free of HIV-related symptoms for years despite continuous replication of HIV in the lymphoid organs that had been seeded during the acute phase of infection. Perhaps somehow the virus tampered with part of the immune system causing it to recognize the virus as a self antigen, or in other words as part of the body so the immune system won't attack it. This would account for the lack of symptoms. Yet, virtually all AIDS patients tested had antibodies against HIV. Cancer patients, I have no doubt also have antibodies against cancer. This suggests a state of only partial tolerance (not 100%).

Despite the body's aggressive immune responses, which are sufficient to clear most viral infections, some HIV invariably escapes. The body's best soldiers in the fight against HIV, certain subsets of killer T cells that recognize HIV, may become depleted or dysfunctional.

In addition, early in the course of HIV infection, people may lose HIV-specific CD4+ T cell responses that normally slow the replication of viruses. Such responses include the secretion of interferons and other antiviral factors, and the orchestration of CD8+ T cells.

Like cancer, for whatever reason the immune system no longer attacks HIV as it should. HIV may cause a multitude of problems but so will anything if your immune system does not attack it, so these problems would normally be nothing serious. Don't let them distract you from finding the source of the trouble.

Cancer does not cause any symptoms because the immune system does not respond to it, but if it's transplanted (like an organ transplant) and rejected it will cause some serious symptoms. Immunosuppressant drugs are necessary with organ transplants because without them the patients' immune system would attack the transplanted organ. The flu-like symptoms of HIV are caused by the immune system responding to the virus and not the virus itself. If those symptoms are absent, that means the immune responses that cause them are absent.

The fact that normal viruses can cause slow viral infections shows that a slow viral infection is more of a condition that can be triggered rather than just an infection.

Vaccines do not always work against slow viruses because the immune system soon develops some degree of tolerance to such viruses. To cure HIV you would need to trigger an immune response against it, but chances are the virus would just trigger tolerance again in a matter of weeks so you would have to reinitiate an immune response every few weeks to cure it. To cure AIDS permanently you would have to find out how the virus triggers tolerance. Once you do you should be able to figure out how to block that from happening and cure AIDS once and for all.

To trigger an immune response attach viral antigens to another type of antigen. This will cause the immune system to attack both antigens. The virus may well cause tolerance to its own antigens in a few weeks but it would not for the other antigen so the next time you inject it, it will still trigger an immune response against the virus. Or it might just be for the other antigen.

Once you figure out how the virus triggers tolerance you should be able to cause tolerance for organ transplants so that immune suppressants would no longer be necessary. This could also cure autoimmune disease and allergies.

In order to figure out how slow viruses cause tolerance write down every thing they do in the body, down to the smallest detail and find out what they all have in common. Search for the common factor.

You will know if your cure works when the patient starts showing symptoms. An AIDS patient will start showing flu-like symptoms and an SSEP patient will come down with the measles.

PART 2

There are 2 main types of tolerance, B cells and T cells. HIV infects T cells so it most likely causes T cell tolerance. T cells develop in the thymus and HIV infects the thymus.

In the thymus, antigen presenting cells present self antigens to the T cells. T cells whose receptors bind to these antigens so tightly that they could attack the cell displaying them are deleted by apoptosis, also known as programmed cell death, which means the cell commits suicide. Or at least we have evidence that indicates that. HIV occasionally infects cells other than CD4+ T cells and may even infect cells that do not contain CD4. I believe the virus might have infected antigen presenting cells causing them to display viral antigens on their surface so any T cells that bind to them will die by apoptosis.

Lack of Co-stimulation

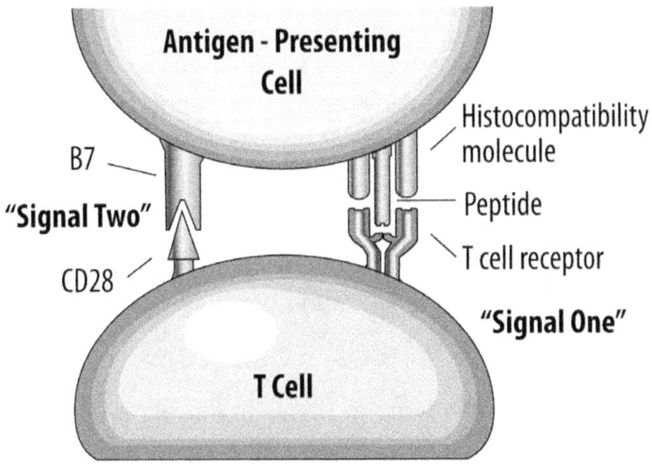

This is called co-stimulation, which is needed to activate T cells. If the T cell fails to receive "signal two," it dies by apoptosis.

Unprimed T cells are cells that have generated an antigen receptor (TCR), but have not yet encountered an antigen.

The binding of a T cell to an antigen-presenting cell (APC)

is by itself not enough to activate that T cell and turn it into an effector cell: one able to, for example, kill the antigen-presenting cell (*CD8⁺ cytotoxic T lymphocytes*), carry out cell-mediated immune reactions (*CD4⁺ Th1 cells*), and provide help to B cells (*CD4⁺ Th2 cells*).

In order to become activated, the T cell would also have to receive a **second signal** from the antigen-presenting cell. This is called **co-stimulation**. Among the most important of these co-stimulators are molecules on the antigen-presenting cell designated **B7** and their ligand (connecting molecule) on the T cell designated **CD28**. The binding of CD28 to B7 provides the second signal needed to activate the T cell.

Although T cells may encounter self antigens in the body, they will not respond unless they receive this second signal. In fact, there is some evidence that the binding of their TCR (signal one) without signal two causes them to self-destruct by apoptosis. Most of the time the cells presenting the body's own antigens fail to provide signal two, and self-tolerance results. If signal 2 is provided the T cell will recognize the antigen as foreign and attack it.

Once HIV infects the lymphoid system there may be so many viral antigens in such close proximity to unprimed T cells that some of the unprimed T cells might bind to them without ever receiving signal 2.

Most of the time the cells presenting the body's own antigens fail to provide signal two, and self-tolerance results. So these cells must go around picking up self antigens from the human body and presenting them to the T cells. They would intentionally not provide signal two in order to cause self tolerance. Self tolerance is necessary because without it our immune systems would attack our own bodies. I wonder if these cells could have picked up cancer or HIV antigens by mistake, thinking that they were self antigens. They would then present HIV antigens to T Cells, as if they were the body's own antigens, without co-stimulation.

PART 3

All slow virus infections have a long latent period after initial infection and before symptoms appear. Why is that?

Perhaps the virus needs time to build up it's antigens in the body in order to cause tolerance. Without this long latent period it wouldn't have the tolerance it needs to become a slow viral infection.

After the flu-like symptoms have passed, a person may remain free of HIV-related symptoms for years despite continuous replication of HIV. How is that possible? Shouldn't the persons' immune system get weak and sick earlier? How can they stay healthy for so long?

Perhaps to begin with the virus only causes a small amount of tolerance so only a small amount of the virus is permitted in the body and over time little by little it causes more and more tolerance until eventually the body is loaded with the virus. This would explain why the virus increases in number so slowly.

Since the immune system recognizes the virus as part of the body it would keep it in check (in the correct proportion). On the other hand, the more viruses there are the more tolerance they cause so the level of tolerance should accelerate over time.

Suppressor T cells

T cells not only require antigen presentation but also co-stimulation for activation. It is now clear that if T cells are not co-stimulated they become anergic. Anergic T cells are live and viable but not functional. Human *in vitro* studies in Professor Lechler's laboratory have shown that anergic T cells act as potent suppressor cells. Data published by the group last year shows that anergic T cells can prolong tolerance in skin grafts in rodents. What is not yet clear is the mechanism underlying this phenomenon.

Once HIV infects the lymphoid system there may be so many viral antigens in such close proximity to unprimed T cells that some of the unprimed T cells might bind directly to them without ever receiving co-stimulation. This theory is probably not what happens since it is relatively safe to assume that a T cell's antigen receptors are closed to antigens unless an antigen presenting cell opens them. It's like a key and a lock. Without the antigen presenting cell it won't fit. It's also a safety mechanism to prevent T cells from binding to just about anything they come across. More likely, because there are so many HIV antigens, certain antigen presenting cells that normally present self antigens may have picked up some of these other antigens by mistake.

This would cause suppressor T cells which would shelter some of the viruses from the immune system. Any extra viruses would be unprotected and would soon be destroyed. That is why some of the viruses remain after the flu-like symptoms and immune response have ended. Over time the virus antigens would cause more and more tolerance so little by little the viruses would increase in number. The more viruses there are the more tolerance they cause so this should accelerate over time. The immune system however would keep the virus numbers in check. This would slow the replication of the virus down, and then of course there are other factors like the breakdown of the antigen filters in the lymph nodes. Since the body keeps the virus in check, the speed of the virus must be entirely dependant on the increasing level of tolerance which could be made possible by the degradation of the immune system.

Elephantiasis

Elephantiasis is caused by a threadlike parasitic worm that makes nests in a person's lymph system. The result is fever, skin lesions, and swelling of the legs and genitalia. Most medications are ineffective against the worm. Not everyone harboring active worms showed overt elephantiasis symptoms and an infection can linger for years or decades before becoming deadly. As far as I can tell, any infection of the lymphoid system has the potential to turn into a slow infection.

Carcinoma: The most common form of cancer arises from the cells forming the skin, the glands (such as the mammary and prostate), the uterus, and the membranes of the respiratory and gastrointestinal tracts; it metastasizes (spreads to other parts of the body) mainly through the lymph vessels. I'm not sure but there might be some connection here. Lymphoma: Malignant tumor of the lymphoid tissue.

In a localized infection immune cells flock to that area. I would assume that suppressor T cells also gather around whatever antigen they are protecting. Another option would be that suppressor cells could just gather around a certain area of the immune system and break the immunological chain of command. The immune system has a chain of signaling molecules like how the nervous system has neurotransmitters. By breaking the chain of communication for a particular antigen, suppressor T cells could end the stimuli for an immune response making the immune system almost blind to that antigen. They act like neuro-inhibitors which inhibit the initiation of a nerve impulse. The more suppressor T cells there are the less of a signal gets through and the less of an immune response you get.

If suppressor T cells are protecting the virus there is the possibility that even the initiation of an immune response might not be able to destroy them since there is already an immune response going on anyway; it's just that the signal is being suppressed or blocked. If such is the case then it might be necessary to kill those suppressor T cells by means of some sort of anti-suppressant T cell medication, but I don't like the idea. Chances are there would always be at least a few of them to shelter some of the viruses. It would be far better to try to figure out some way of preventing the virus from causing tolerance. This along with the immune response should be able to wipe them out.

How animals tolerate pregnancy without rejecting the fetus is only partially understood. Current theories are that there is a barrier that masks the fetal antigens and that the maternal immune system is suppressed. If suppressor T cells are involved in the tolerance of a fetus, organ transplants, and skin grafts, people with such conditions should not take anti-suppressor T cell medication.

Tolerant T cells given to an animal can protect that animal from graft rejection provided the graft contains the same antigens to which the T cells are tolerant. The tolerance in this case is temporary and only maintained by the presence of the tolerant T cells. I read that they caused tolerance for a kidney transplant by transplanting some of the donor's bone marrow. Bone marrow is part of the immune system since bone marrow produces white blood cells. Perhaps the transplantation of lymphoid tissue would have a similar effect in order to cause tolerance for grafts and transplants.

Suppressor T cells are not well understood. They are generally thought to regulate the immune response by turning it off when an antigen is no longer present. I disagree with this theory. An immune response is stimulated by antigens. Once those antigens are absent so is the stimuli, so the immune response should end all on its own. I wonder if the suppressor T cells stop the immune system from responding by somehow ending the stimuli, perhaps by breaking the chain of immunological communication; this thought was the origin of the theory you read earlier, the one using neurotransmitters as an example.

HIV disrupts the network of signaling molecules that normally regulates a person's immune response. That is an awfully complex task for a virus. Sounds more like something suppressor T cells would do. Researchers have shown in cell cultures that

CD4+ T cells can be turned off by activation signals from HIV that leaves them unable to respond to further immune stimulation. This inactivated state is known as anergy. If the cultures did not contain any antigen presenting cells to provide co-stimulation then this would probably happen. The activation signals are probably just viral antigens binding directly to the T Cells without co-stimulation. This is based on the theory that T cells' antigen receptors can bind directly to viral antigens without antigen presenting cells to present them.

In another theory, the cell cultures would have to have been contaminated with "self antigen presenting cells" which would have presented HIV antigens to the T cells as self antigens, without co-stimulation. The idea is that antigen presenting cells can act in different modes of operation. Sometimes they present antigens as foreign so that the immune system will attack them and sometimes they present antigens as self antigens so that the immune system will be tolerant of them. Since unprimed T cells and antigen presenting cells work closely together they can be found closely together in the body and it is quite likely that some antigen presenting cells were added to the culture along with the T cells.

If suppressor T cells were produced then they could have provided the activation signals, and suppressed the CD4+ T cells, leaving them unable to respond to further immune stimulation. This inactivated state is known as anergy.

Suppressor T cells are also important in the maintenance of self-tolerance, preventing self-directed T cells that avoid clonal deletion in the thymus from mounting immune responses against the body itself. Suppressor T cells usually carry CD8 receptors, whereas most T helper cells carry CD4 receptors.

That means HIV would be less likely to infect suppressor T cells and they'll live longer.

Suppressor T cells may also protect us from allergic reactions as in the case of induced tolerance. **Induced tolerance** is tolerance to external antigens that has been created by deliberately manipulating the immune system. Its' importance is to protect us from unpleasant and even dangerous allergic reactions to such things as food (e.g. peanuts), insect stings, grass pollen (hay fever) and to avoid graft rejection.

This is probably the kind of tolerance involved in HIV. It is an introduced antigen after all. It is possible that the immune system might have mistaken HIV antigens for harmless allergens and thus developed tolerance to them. Cancer antigens on the other hand, look a great deal like self antigens so cancer is probably a case of self tolerance and the exact same type of tolerance seems to be involved in both cancer and HIV.

Technically, induced tolerance is tolerance to external antigens so HIV is not a case of induced tolerance. HIV is an internal antigen like an organ transplant. Organ transplants are foreign substances that have been introduced into the body in the same way that allergens are external antigens that have entered into the body. It may be that in the end there is no difference between induced tolerance and self tolerance.

I just realized something. Allergens like pollen normally enter our lungs and tuberculosis infects the lungs. The immune system could have become tolerant of tuberculosis the same as it would an allergen. The fact that tuberculosis can last for years shows that it is not an ordinary infection. When the body's normal defenses cannot prevent or overcome a disease, it is often treated with chemotherapy [drugs]. Chemotherapy is used to treat cancer, HIV, and tuberculosis. To be effective against tuberculosis, chemotherapy must be continued for one to two years. Definitely not an ordinary infection. Perhaps this data may prove to be far more useful than in just infections of the lymphoid system. Although, now that I think about it, I remember there are lymph nodes located in the lungs as well.

Supporting evidence

Vaccines: In general, gram to milligram quantities of protein antigens are needed to elicit an antibody response in a laboratory animal. This range, which may differ from antigen to antigen and from species to species, is called the "window of immunogenicity." Too much or too little antigen may induce tolerance rather than an active response for the given antigen. ~sounds like my theory of AIDS causing tolerance. ~The **Animal Welfare Information Center (AWIC)**, part of the National Agricultural Library (NAL) of the U.S. Department of Agriculture (USDA). http://www.nal.usda.gov/awic/pubs/antibody/overview.htm

The ratio of helper T cells to suppressor T cells is a useful determinant of immune function. If the ratio is too low, immunodeficiency is present. For example, AIDS is characterized by a very low ratio of helper T cells to suppressor T cells. If the ratio is too high, allergies or autoimmune disorders such as rheumatoid arthritis and lupus are often present. Both high and low ratios have been found in chronic fatigue syndrome. ~ Alternative medicine: The definitive guide by the Burton Goldberg Group page, 147

Suppressor T cells are also called regulatory T cells because they regulate the immune system.

According to the encyclopedia, Wikipedia, experimental evidence from mouse models suggests that some pathogens may have evolved to manipulate regulatory T cells (also known as suppressor T cells) to immunosuppress the host and so potentiate their own survival. For example, regulatory T cell activity has been reported to increase in several infectious contexts, such as retroviral infections and various parasitic infections including Leishmania and malaria. ~As stated at the beginning of this book, HIV is a retrovirus. ~Wikipedia, Article: Regulatory T cell

Web Site: http://en.wikipedia.org/wiki/Suppressor_T_cells

HIV actually stands for Human Immunodeficiency Virus. Even the name, HIV stands for a deficiency of the immune system.

CHAPTER 2

The Solution

Before you can treat something, you have to know what the problem is. Now that we know what's wrong we can fix it.

There are 2 main options as far as I can tell. Either stop the virus from causing tolerance or undo the tolerance the virus has created.

To undo the tolerance the virus has created would, in all likelihood, undo the tolerance to our own bodies. Any attempt to suppress the production of CD8+ T cells that might later turn into suppressor T cells, prevent them from interrupting the signaling processes of the immune system, or kill off the suppressor T cells themselves and our immune systems would end up attacking our own bodies. This leaves the first option which is to stop the virus from causing tolerance which is the actual problem.

Again, the problem is that antigens could bind directly to unprimed T cells without co-stimulation. This is the old theory.

Perhaps an herbalist or maybe a druggist might be able to

come up with something that would affect the lymph system. We have drugs to suppress the immune system. An immune stimulant, perhaps. One that would be able to stimulate the production of "antigen presenting cells," for instance? It would certainly decrease the likelihood of a lack of co-stimulation. If we had more antigen presenting cells we'd have more antigens being presented with co-stimulation and less antigens binding to T cells on their own.

We could decrease the amount of viral antigens in the body. Decreasing the amount of viral antigens has already been tried which means, undoubtedly that the answer lies in increasing co-stimulation. Also, of course, we cannot remove all cancer antigens.

We all produce at least a few cancer cells throughout our lives, but normally our immune systems fight them off. People who get cancer are not under an extreme assault of cancer antigens like how an AIDS patient gets too many HIV antigens which causes tolerance, so a cancer patient shouldn't be tolerant of cancer. They should be able to fight off the cancer like the rest of us, but since they cannot, they probably suffer from a lack of "antigen presenting cells." Without enough antigen presenting cells to present the antigens properly some antigens could bind directly to the T cells on their own. The simplest cure would be to correct this lack.

But there is no evidence that they have a lack of antigen presenting cells, it sounds like it would be a rare genetic condition, and often people get cancer after coming into contact with something else, a carcinogen, or when they don't take care of themselves or later in life or something else so the root cause doesn't seem like it would be a lack of antigen presenting cells. There's no reason for all of these different people to have such a condition.

If what is actually happening is that antigen presenting cells are presenting HIV or cancer antigens as self antigens then the theory of there being a lack of antigen presenting cells is without foundation. Also, increasing the number of antigen presenting cells could mean that more antigens would be presented as self antigens so this could actually make things worse. Although whether it makes this better or worse would depend on how increasing their numbers would affect the ratio of the antigens they present as foreign to the antigens they present as self antigens.

Another Theory

Another theory would be that you could either get rid of the viral antigens or prevent the antigen presenting cells from picking them up in the first place. If you can't get rid of all the viral antigens, then if you could just stop the antigen presenting cells from accidently picking them up, you could correct the tolerance.

As stated before antigen presenting cells have two modes of operation. Sometimes they present antigens as self antigens and sometimes they present antigens as foreign so that the immune system will attack them.

Substances that boost the activity of antigen presenting cells are often polysaccharides found in certain mushrooms. These substances boost the likelihood that antigen presenting cells will present antigens as foreign which is the second function.

They probably do this by being very noticeable foreign substances in the body. This would stimulate the immune system and the immune system would increase the second function of antigen presenting cells (as well as the activity of other immune cells) because of the foreign substance.

It may be counter intuitive to boost the activity of cells that could present HIV antigens as self antigens but remember, we are only increasing the second function and in the past people have used things that boost the activity of antigen presenting cells to help fight off disease, and it seems to work.

Putting the immune system into this state causes antigen presenting cells to be more likely to present antigens as foreign which means they will be less likely to pick them up as self antigens.

This is actually just what you want.

If you could stop the antigen presenting cells from picking up HIV antigens instead of self antigens then you could end the tolerance. However that is not what happens here.

This only makes antigen presenting cells more likely to present HIV as a foreign antigen so it only makes antigen presenting cells present HIV as foreign more often.

Unfortunately, I doubt that polysaccharides from mushrooms would be able to overcome the tolerance by themselves, although they certainly would help.

The real benefit here doesn't come from antigen presenting cells presenting foreign antigens as self antigens a little less often. Just a few antigens wouldn't matter very much.

The real benefit comes from the antigen presenting cells triggering a small immune response. The immune response (or the antibodies) could get rid of a fair amount of antigens so this actually does remove some of the viral antigens in a round about way.

"Whoops," when I mentioned not being able to decrease the amount of viral antigens I was only thinking of antiviral therapy which reduces the viral burden, but there are other ways of decreasing the amount of antigens, so we could still try decreasing the viral antigens in the body. The fewer antigens there are, the less likely they will be presented as self antigens so decreasing the viral antigens is still a good idea. In order to do this however, we would first need to know a bit more about the lymph system.

Lymph System: There is twice as much lymph fluid in our bodies as there is blood, and we have twice as many lymph vessels as blood vessels. Our cells are located in a sea of lymph, a pale fluid. Oxygen and sugar are transported from the blood vessels to nourish the cells via the lymphatic fluid. The lymph carries nutrients to the parts of the body where the blood cannot go and carries away wastes, emptying it into the bloodstream.

The lymph system, which is throughout the body, is the "highway" by which wastes are transported from the cells to the blood and from there to the colon and kidneys for elimination. The lymph system acts as a mini sewer system because one of its main jobs is to remove cellular wastes and toxins from the body.

Like the cardiovascular system, the lymphatic system is made up of channels or vessels, valves and filters (nodes). Unlike the bloodstream, however, there is no pump like the heart. Instead, the lymphatic fluid is forced through the system by the action of the muscles and breathing.

The lymph system becomes particularly active during times of illness (such as the flu), when the nodes (particularly at the neck) visibly swell with collected waste products.

Lymph fluid is supposed to be clear but if the lymph system fails to function properly it can go from watery to milk-like to yogurt to cottage cheese. Thickened, gel-like lymph fluid will not flow as it should and it can become sluggish or even stagnant. This is what happens when the lymph system becomes congested. If you've ever had a congested, stuffy head then you probably have some idea of what's going on in the lymph system. When the lymphatic system becomes congested, the lymphatic system's drainage becomes blocked.

The **nodes filter lymph** fluid and **remove dangerous impurities** such as dead red blood cells, millions of debris-laden white blood cells, chemicals, and dyes but if blocked, the lymph nodes also become storage points for waste.

Conclusions

With this many antigens in the body, it's no wonder why antigen presenting cells might pick up viral antigens instead of self antigens. It would be next to impossible for antigen presenting cell not to pick them up accidently.

It could be that antigen presenting cells are always picking up antigens at random in the body and causing tolerance to them. The majority of antigens in our bodies are self antigens so the majority of tolerance would be self tolerance. The majority of disease causing antigens would be picked up in the lymph system because that is where toxins antigens and wastes tend to accumulate.

This could make it look like antigen presenting cells just pick up antigens for self presentation in the lymph system when in fact it's just because that's where the highest concentration of antigens are. They could actually pick them up just about anywhere in the body.

If disease antigens got into the lymph system (or in the body in general) under ordinary circumstances they would not have a high enough density to cause much tolerance and the disease would be destroyed by the immune system.

People who are prone to cancer probably suffer from poor circulation in their lymph system which would cause a build-up of cancer antigens, and not a lack of antigen presenting cells as I had suspected earlier. There is a lack of antigens being presented with co-stimulation, but only in comparison to the number of antigens being presented without co-stimulation.

Sometimes when a tumor is removed the cancer comes back worse than it was before. The reason is that when doctors remove the tumor they also, unavoidably remove some of the lymph nodes. The lymph vessels are supposed to remove wastes and antigens but once they have been removed or severed they can no longer do that.

Since the highest concentration of cancer antigens would

be immediately around the tumor, it is likely that the highest level of tolerance would be immediately around the tumor as well. The highest levels of suppressor T cells for the cancer would also be around the tumor because that is where they get produced.

It is possible that cancer only spreads to where its antigens have spread first. Carcinoma spreads mainly through the lymph system and other types of cancer spread mainly from the area immediately around the tumor.

If any cancer cells suddenly moved away from the tumor and out of this tolerant area, they would probably be destroyed by the immune system. You don't often see a tumor in a shape that has a lot of surface area and even HIV has a tendency to build up in little clusters in the lymph nodes. It is not spread evenly throughout the body because of the immune system. Even when there is relatively little HIV in the blood there can be a great deal of HIV bundled up in the lymph system, just like a tumor.

This is not just because it gets stuck in the lymph nodes' filtering systems. It's because any HIV that's away from the dense cloud of antigens gets destroyed more easily.

The degradation of the immune system

If the flu can make the nodes swell just think of what AIDS can do. Even early in disease, HIV actively replicates within the lymph nodes and related organs, where large amounts of the virus become trapped in networks of specialized cells called follicular dendritic cells (FDCs). These cells have long, tentacle-like extensions that act like flypaper, trapping invading pathogens, like HIV, and holding them there until B cells come along to start an immune response.

Over a period of years, even when low levels of HIV are readily detectable in the blood, significant amounts of the virus accumulate in the lymphoid tissue, both within infected cells and bound to FDCs.

This leads to the **Breakdown of the lymph node architecture.** Ultimately, with chronic cell activation and secretion of inflammatory cytokines, the fine and complex inner structure of the lymph node breaks down and is replaced by scar tissue. Without this structure, cells in the lymph node cannot communicate and the immune system cannot function properly. This scarring also reduces the ability of the immune system to replenish itself following antiretroviral therapy which reduces the viral burden.

The lymph nodes in the lungs of people who live in large smog-laden cities are often completely black from the soot that they filter from the air. ~I wonder if there's a way to clear up the nodes.

Excessive antigens clogging the lymph system is the real problem and even though increasing the activity of antigen presenting cells would help, clearing the lymph system is vital and absolutely necessary.

CHAPTER 3

What Can Be Done To Clear The Lymph System?

To keep it clear, you need to increase its drainage capacity or reduce its intake of toxins - through diet, stress reduction, exercise and deep breathing.

This might sound mild for treating AIDS, but remember we're treating cancer here too so be patient, and this same stuff goes for AIDS anyway. These seemingly weak treatments can be very powerful for those whom they apply to or for those who are specifically in need of these things.

Stress depresses the immune system. Stress hormones inhibit white blood cell function and formation as well as cause the thymus to shrink (involute). Emotions have a tremendous impact on immune function. Whenever you stress anything it wears it out. You need your rest. Stress has the opposite effect. When you're stressed all of your energy goes into using up your most immediate energy reserves and none into recuperation.

Exercise, such as taking walks helps to move the lymph fluid. The lymphatic fluid, which is twice the volume of the blood, normally circulates throughout the body once a day. Exercise can increase lymphatic flow threefold (or more with extreme exercise), but if you're sick don't over do it. Swinging your arms is also recommended.

Deep breathing is important, because the lymph collected throughout the body drains into the blood through two ducts situated at the base of the neck, the main one being the thoracic duct, and breathing drives this action. "If you take a deep breath and exhale deeply, you're massaging the thoracic duct upward into the neck so that the fluid flows generously," a certain Dr. Lemole explains. "This duct empties the lymph into the veins, where it becomes part of the blood plasma. From there the lymph returns to the liver for metabolization, and finally to the kidneys for filtering."

Diet: A person with a weak lymphatic system should eliminate all wheat and dairy products from their diet. These foods become quite pasty in the body and can easily clog the lymphatic system. Too much sugar will lead to lowered white blood cell activity. Nutrient deficiency is the most common cause of low immunity. If there's a deficiency of a nutrient, there will be a deficiency in whatever your body normally uses that nutrient for.

Stomach

Another thing having to do with diet is the way you process food. If your stomach acid is not acidic enough your stomach may not be able to break down food properly and undigested food will build up in your intestines. Bacteria will then produce extra acid to break down the food and, as the food putrefies, the acid will penetrate your intestinal wall, and then lower the pH of your entire body thereby creating a more disease friendly environment.

Not everyone has too little stomach acid but for those who do, a common cure is to drink apple cider vinegar since it can raise the acid levels of your stomach.

Another way to prevent undigested food from entering your intestines is to chew your food more thoroughly. Your stomach acid and enzymes can only digest the food that they come into contact with and they cannot come into contact with the inside of large hunks of food. If the food is in small enough pieces then all of it can get wet and all of it can get digested so either chew your food or put it in the blender.

Constipation

In order to keep toxins and waste products from building up in your body it is very important that nothing interferes with your ability to eliminate waste. If you are constipated, you cannot eliminate waste products properly. You see, some of the wastes from the lymph system are transported to the intestines via the lacteals, which is the part of the lymph system that empties into the small intestines. The waste then passes into the large intestine for elimination. When the intestinal walls are impacted the lymph system retains the waste. At this point toxins will begin to build up in the lymph system and the prolific number of lymph nodes in the abdominal region will also become storage points for waste.

Retaining waste products is a lot like retaining water in your tissues. The tissues become bloated and this interferes with intestinal muscular contractions, thereby worsening the constipation. Intestinal contractions are what moves the poop along and are necessary for proper bowel function.

Even if you do not think that you're constipated, if your lymph system is congested it's very important that you eliminate all the waste from your body that you can. The American diet often lacks fiber. The easiest way to fix this situation is either to drink hot prune juice or eat prunes. They'll make your bowels move, they're natural, and they're good for you. Fiber should be a part of your diet and you should eat it regularly.

Exercises that either bend or flex the abdominal region can also be helpful for moving poop along. When you move your abdomen you move your bowels. You don't need difficult exercise. Movement is all that's necessary. Even walking (or marching) will help. It also helps to move the lymph fluid in the intestinal area. You could even bend your abdomen while setting down just by rocking back and forth.

Water

Your bladder and kidneys are also important for eliminating waste so be sure to drink plenty of water, don't strain your kidneys, and don't hold your pee. Holding your pee is like holding your poop (or constipation). When you hold your pee it prevents your kidneys from doing their job and pollutes the body. Dehydration has a similar polluting effect and water will flush you out.

Water is good for you but drinking too much water during meals dilutes the stomach acid and enzymes and forces the pancreas to overwork so you might want to drink a little throughout the day. Keep all things in moderation.

Liver

Another important filtration device is the liver. The liver filters out toxins, poison and viruses from your blood, so take care of your liver. That means avoid alcohol. Alcohol hardens the liver. Alcohol is a medicine and you're not supposed to get high on it. If you don't think the liver is important just remember you'd die without it.

The coffee enema is a popular liver cleanser. It causes the liver to produce more bile, opens the bile ducts and causes the bile to flow. The liver can then dump many of its toxins into the bile and get rid of them within minutes. For a less drastic course of action, consult your local health food store. Just about every health food store carries something specifically formulated for your liver.

For more information on the subject of the coffee enema see A Liver Cleanser "S.A. Wilsons Therapy Blend Coffee" web site: http://www.sawilsons.com/liver.htm based upon Dr. Gerson's work. More information is available in his book: A Cancer Therapy, Results of Fifty Cases.

By the way, while we're on the subject of diet; drinking coffee has a very different effect from the coffee enema. Drinking coffee stimulates the body and when you're sick you need your rest. The coffee enema, if administered properly, will not do that.

If you're sick don't drink coffee. Its' ability to stimulate the adrenals mimics the effects of stress. Prolonged use of coffee mimics the effects of prolonged stress. Like cigarettes and alcohol it takes a while to cause permanent or long term symptoms. There's a good reason why most parents won't let young children drink coffee. I don't think coffee will kill you but I know it won't do you any good (especially when you're sick) and chances are so do you.

Spleen

The thymus and spleen are also considered part of the immune system so you might want to do some research on those as well. The spleen is similar to the lymph nodes, except that it filters blood instead of lymph. If you have leukemia or a long term blood illness you should take care of your blood filters to keep it clean.

Celery seed has been used to treat certain diseases of the liver and spleen as well as colds, flu, water retention, and poor digestion. Today, celery seed is used primarily as a diuretic, increasing urine output to help the body to get rid of excess water and to clean out the body of its wastes, especially uric acid in the joints (as in the case of gout).

The healing properties of celery seed are in the volatile oil, which acts as an antiseptic. In the urinary system, the oil helps clean out the organs that carry urine.

Celery seed is also suggested for treating arthritis and gout, and to help reduce muscle spasms, calm nerves, and reduce inflammation. AIDS patients often have inflamed lymph nodes. Preventing inflammation helps to prevent them from braking down. (*See the section entitled "the degradation of the immune system"*).

A Bad Habit

A lady that my mother takes care of (Nila) agreed to read my book and let me know what she thought. After reading the part about water she just quit drinking soda pop all together and she used to drink at least 6 cans a day because, when she was little, her mother never let her drink soda except on her birthday. She knew that soda was bad for her, but after reading how important water was she was afraid of what might happen to her if she didn't stop drinking soda pop so she had to quit. Now she drinks a lot of water instead.

About a month later she saw a soda pop advertisement on television and she had to have one. The next day, she bought some soda, took one sip, spit it out, and put the rest away in the refrigerator. She said it tasted terrible carbonated and she had to let the carbonation out of it in order to drink it. Then it tasted fine. She sipped it over a period of days. I think it was her body letting her know that it wasn't good for her and that's why it tasted bad. She drank it anyway because she needed something besides water. I think the reason why it tasted fine uncarbonated was because her body didn't remember soda being uncarbonated and so it didn't recognize what it was.

About 2 months after she quit, her fingers started turning brown. It scared her because her fiancée's whole body and even his irises had turned a golden brown before he died. She admired his beautiful golden eyes but it wasn't natural. She asked my mother to ask me what to do. I remembered a story I had heard. A man had been a heavy smoker for many years and right after he quit smoking he got lung cancer. The theory was that the body stores toxins and right after he quit smoking his body quit storing the toxins and they all came rushing out and gave him cancer and that's what killed him. Nilas' fiancée had died of pancreatic cancer and his skin was brown because his liver was going out. The liver is what processes the toxins. Nila found a mole on her arm with seriated purple, light brown, and pink coloring around it and was scared that it might be skin cancer.

If she drank some soda again, just a little, her body might get a taste of it and start actively storing the toxins away again where they can't do any more harm. Right now they were overwhelming her system. I told my mother to pick out a flavor of soda that she didn't like and give her one can a day for 3 days and then one every other day until her fingers got better. I also told her to tell Nila the 'smoker story' so she would know what was going on. My mother picked out diet soda because that's what Nila always used to drink and that's what her body was adjusted to. but she didn't forget to get a flavor of diet soda that Nila didn't like. We can't have her getting addicted again. Nila didn't like drinking it, tastes terrible, but she did because she understood that, that was her medicine now. The smoker story scared her. I'm worried too. I think we got it in time but I won't know until later.

Even if she did get skin cancer it is possible for her to un-get cancer. Everyone has at least a few cancer cells in their body. Her body always did just fine with fighting off the cancer cells before. If we can get her body into the same condition as it was before, it will respond to the cancer the same as it did before and it will clear up, but it's not just her body. It's her immune system and a state of tolerance and clearing up a toxin congested immune system and then ending the tolerance would probably be one of the last things to get back to normal. I still think we got it in time though because her fingers seemed to have cleared up just a hair and then stayed the same by the time I found out about it. Even if the toxins aren't getting any worse the tolerance could, so it's good that I found out about it when I did. The progression of a disease is not up to the germ. Its fate is determined by your immune system.

If you've been a really heavy smoker for years and years and then you just quit for a month to give your body time to figure out that it's not good for you without a single cigarette in between, you had better pick out a brand of cigarettes that you really don't like and set a schedule to take them just to give your body a taste. Nicotine patches won't work because your body has gotten used to having the toxins in your lungs. If you just started smoking then maybe you can quit right now, and you should. If the smog of large cities can turn the lymph nodes of a person's lungs black then just think about what cigarettes can do and then think about what would happen if you had a condition in your immune system. But remember, the body can even become dependant on coffee, withdraw symptoms aren't good for you, and your body can't stand a shock. It takes time to adjust so do all things in moderation.

On Nilas' third day on soda pop, the brown on her fingers disappeared all the way back down to her fingernails and I found out later that before, it had gone all the way up to the palm of her right hand. I didn't expect anything so dramatic.

The previous day gave no indication that she was getting any better. The body takes time to react and switch gears. Also the skin around her mole got lighter and the mole itself got darker. Before, the skin around the mole was brown and purple and a little pink. I guess it was cancer after all or it wouldn't have changed like that. Nila is happy now and happy too that she doesn't have to drink her soda pop tomorrow. We're weaning her off of it. I think she'll be just fine.

The super-diseases of the past such as the plague, typhoid fever, and rabies that terrorized the world are now virtually non-existent in civilized countries. It is possible that our modern super-diseases may be even easier to get rid of, but only if you direct your efforts directly into fixing what's actually wrong.

Fourth day: All the coloring around the mole has almost completely disappeared. It's almost undetectable. The mole itself is much darker and a little smaller in diameter and just a hair taller. My mother said it's amazing. I spoke to Nila on the phone today. I told her that I thought it probably was cancer, but it is possible to un-get cancer. She said "O yeah, I know. I knew some people that had cancer, but it went away."

5th Day: The mole is completely gone and there's only a hair of brown under the tips of her fingernails. She'll still have to take a can of soda every few days for a while though.

The Lymph fluid

Manual lymphatic drainage (MLD) is an important part of the treatment of lymphedema. To be effective in treating lymphedema, it is important to use the correct technique. The massage is designed to move the excess fluid away from the swollen areas so that it can drain away normally. Manual lymphatic drainage differs from an ordinary massage and since this is a specialized form of massage, it should be given only by a trained therapist. I read that skin brushing is also an excellent way to move your excess lymph fluid.

Vibratory machines: The "Lymphstar Pro" is a machine based on vibrational energy technology and harmonics. Current price: between $2,600 and $3,000. It is more for an alternative health care professional that has a private practice and sees many patients than for an individual. A simple vibratory device might be best for you. A vibrating back massager that you could take to bed with you, for instance. They even make vibrating chairs.

You've got to keep your fluids moving. In men the nodes, in the crease of the groin, are the primary channel for release of accumulated lymph from the prostrate. In women the axillary nodes, located in the arm pit, are the primary channel for releasing accumulated lymph from the breasts. This is probably why there is so much breast cancer. If the axillary nodes get plugged up then they will not be able to remove the antigens and prostate cancer is one of the most common types of cancer in men.

Flexitouch® System

The Flexitouch system (Tactile Systems Technology, Minneapolis, MN) consists of an electronic controller device and garments that fits over the trunk and upper and lower extremities of the body, with chambers that sequentially inflate and deflate at 1 to 3 second intervals to help move your lymph fluid in the right direction.

It is used in the treatment of lymphedema and edema, but it is only available with a prescription. The Flexitouch® Lymphedema System is UL classified and has FDA marketing clearance and proven more effective than self-administered MLD (Manual Lymphatic Drainage).

Infrared heat lamp

For people who are old or obese, have trouble exercising and have edema in their legs (retaining fluid and waste products in their tissues) it may help to have a far infrared heat lamp pointed at the legs, tumor, or elsewhere.

The infra-red heat lamp helps the blood to circulate and once the fluids start circulating, it will help to clean out the built up waste products in the legs. Once this waste is removed from the legs waste products from the upper body can settle down in the legs and they can be removed too.

An Infrared Heat Lamp has a special effect which an ordinary heating pad is said not to have. It is effective when deep heating of body tissue is desired. An ordinary heating pad cannot heat deep inside of your tissues without burning the outside of your skin, but an infrared light can penetrate your skin and heat both the inside and the outside relatively evenly, without burning you.

Infrared Light Therapy works by increasing the local circulation of blood, lymph and the activity of the nervous system. A therapy lamp can decrease painful edema, reduces pain in joints, muscles, bones, and relax tense muscles. They actually make infrared therapy lamps designed specifically for this purpose.

Such a lamp could be used to increase the circulation around tumors or make swollen lymph nodes go down.

Alzheimer's: People with Alzheimer's have built up protein wastes in the brain. Such a lamp could even be used to increase the circulation of cerebrospinal fluid in the back to help to remove the protein plaques located in the brain. Spinal fluid acts as the brains lymph fluid to keep it clean. You may want to have several lamps along the spine where cerebrospinal fluid may empty its wastes into the lymph fluid. Cerebral fluid can be clear but it can also become cloudy, just like lymph fluid. It circulates nutrients filtered from the blood to the brain as well as carrying wastes away from the brain.

Some have suggested that the flow of CSF along the cranial nerves and spinal nerve roots allows it into the lymphatic channels; this flow may play a substantial role in CSF re-absorption (or draining). ~Wikipedia article "Cerebrospinal fluid" Warning: warm you spine, don't point lamp directly on brain.

A vibrating bed or pad under your back when you sleep could be used in place of an infrared heat lamp. Because this could be used when you sleep for 8 hours maybe it would be much more effective than only an hour or two in a vibrating chair. Rocking back and forth when you sit and bending your spine can also help to move the spinal fluid.

Clearing out the lymph fluid could also make it easier for the cerebral spinal fluid to empty out into the lymph system. It couldn't do that very well if it was congested. In fact, a congested lymph system could even be what's causing the problem for some people.

Multiple sclerosis (MS): Whatever works for Alzheimer's may also work for MS. Recently they have discovered that the brain has its own immune system and they think that in MS the immune system could be at fault. If the cerebral fluid, which is the equivalent of lymph fluid, is congested then it could cause the immune system to malfunction.

Proper diet and exercise might help but it's probably not going to be enough to treat cancer and it definitely will not be enough for AIDS. More is needed, so here is a list of agents you could take to boost the activity of antigen presenting cells. There are many items other than the ones listed so you might want to do your own research.

First the fine print: We increase the activity of antigen presenting cells because it helps to stimulate a small immune response and counteracts tolerance. However, even though this would help, unclogging the lymph system is what you've got to do because that is the actual problem. Things that would help with this will be mentioned in the following lists.

Fine print on Immunostimulants: Immunostimulants are medicine, not candy. Most of the items mentioned here are not prescription so they should be fairly safe. Just remember that it is even possible to over-dose on vitamins if you over do it.

Stimulating the immune system can be a good thing as long as it's not overdone since over stimulation can theoretically lead to an over active immune system and autoimmune disease.

People have been using immune stimulants against cancer and AIDS with some success, but it does not seem to be enough to cure the disease. Clearing the lymph system is a necessity.

Using immune stimulants against AIDS is however, controversial since the immune system is already largely exhausted and over stimulation of the immune system can lead to immune system exhaustion.

However if the immune system is actually being suppressed then it probably isn't being over stimulated and an HIV patient could take just as many immune-stimulants as a normal person. However this has not been proven.

I do not recommend over stimulating the immune system, but some immune stimulants might also have helpful lymph cleansing effects so you must make your own decisions in this regard. It's dangerous to take chances, but it's also dangerous not to.

List 1:
Agents for boosting the activity of antigen presenting cells

Mushrooms

beta-glucan A type of polysaccharide (string of sugar molecules) obtained from several types of mushrooms. It is being studied as a treatment for cancer and as an immune system stimulant.

lentinan A beta-glucan (a type of polysaccharide) from the mushroom Lentinus edodes (**shiitake mushroom**). It has been studied in Japan as a treatment for cancer. Shiitake is pronounced 'she talk eee'.

Coriolus Mushroom Commonly known as the "**turkey tail**" in North America, *Coriolus versicolor* (and *Trametes versicolor*), it is used in both traditional herbalism and modern clinical practice. Coriolus polysaccharides have been shown to stimulate the **antigen-presenting cell** function of macrophages and, consequently, to stimulate overall immune function. Several studies have also reported the ability of Coriolus polysaccharides to enhance in vitro proliferation of T and B lymphocytes, and to enhance the cytotoxic activity of Natural Killer cells. These polysaccharides are not affected by the digestive process and are therefore effective when used orally.

The reishi mushroom Also known as (Ganoderma lucidum) - Lingzhi - or Ling Zhi. Reishi is a popular Chinese mushroom. The most attractive character of this kind of medicinal fungus is its effect on the immune system and anti-tumor activities. Large numbers of studies have shown that reishi modulates many components of the immune system such as the **antigen-presenting cells**, NK cells, and T and B lymphocytes.

High quality Reishi extracts, according to clinical studies (Kupin 1992, Yang 1996), will increase levels of T-cell counts, CD4 to CD8 ratios, cytokine IL2, complement C3, immunoglobulin G, stimulate the formation of antibodies, lower levels of T-suppressor cells, increase appetite, improve vigor and shorten recovery time.

Reishi can be used long term, but as a general statement, it is not appropriate for use with autoimmune conditions. It acts as an immune system stimulant for some areas of immune function and a modulator for others. It also lowers levels of T-suppressor cells that would normally stop immune attacks.

This might be good news if you have cancer or AIDS but if you have arthritis and your level of suppressor T cells goes down, then there will be fewer of them to stop your immune system from attacking your bones. Something that could modulate the immune response would probably be far better for something like arthritis. An immune modulator is something that helps the body to regulate its own immune system. In theory, if an old persons' immune system stopped attacking their bones (as in arthritis) then the bones might be able to heal and could even get stronger.

List 2:
Items to help with lymph drainage

Maitake mushroom powder is known mostly for supporting proper immune function, which assists in maintaining healthy glandular function and lymph drainage. Maitake contains complex polysaccharides which are among the most potent polysaccharides found in any mushroom or herb. Beta-D-glucan, the primary polysaccharide in Maitake, is well absorbed when taken orally and is being researched for its ability to prevent or treat cancer and as a treatment for HIV infection.

Anything that improves any part of the lymph system will, in a round about way, help with proper lymph drainage. In fact, anything that helps any part of your body is likely to help the rest of it. It's all connected after all, so some of the items in these lists might fit into more than just one category, like the Maitake mushroom for example. Some of these agents perform more than just one function and since the Maitake mushroom contains polysaccharides, you know it would also fit into list number one.

Lymphagogue: An agent which promotes an increase of fluid in the lymph-channels thereby increasing the flow of lymph. An agent which promotes lymph circulation and movement of interstitial fluids. **Lymphagogue**: Herbs or other agents that promote or increases lymph production or lymph flow.

Lymphatic botanicals

Botanicals that can assist the lymphatic system in clearing congestion and accumulated fluids or wastes in the tissues, may reduce fibrocystic pathology. By assisting in the removal of excessive fluids, lymphatics may prevent stagnation and cyst formation in the breasts.

Lymphagogue botanicals (lymph movers) include:

Phytolacca americana, {Pokeweed} also known as *P. de-*

candra (poke root)

Iris versicolor (Iris) Blue flag, Poison flag

Ceanothus americanus (New Jersey tea), sometimes referred to as red root, but there's more than one plant called red root.

Galium aparine (Cleavers or bedstraw)

The strongest of which seems to be poke root, but as far as I know, it is not available without a prescription. You still might be able to get poke root mixed in with other products though. It is dangerous if taken long term. There is a thin line between drugs and herbs... but as far as I know, no one's ever found it yet.

General circulatory tonics such as *Capsicum annum* **(cayenne peppers)** may improve the activity of other botanicals. In Europe, cayenne was used to reduce swollen lymph glands caused by tuberculosis. Increasing the circulation causes excess fluid to leave the swollen area. Pepper spray works so well it can turn your face red (not recommended). **Prickly ash bark** may be used in a way that is similar to cayenne and, although it is slower acting, it also has a stimulating effect on the lymphatic system, circulation and mucous membranes. **Stillingia root** acts primarily on the lymphatic and secretory systems and **wild indigo root** has been used effectively to treat enlarged and inflamed lymph glands.

Celery seed extract is a diuretic and it can also be used to clean out the body. When you take lymphagogues, your body may need to get rid of a lot of wastes from your lymph system so you may want to drink a lot of water at this time to help flush yourself out. A diuretic like celery seed helps the water to do its job. Celery seed also really helps to clean excessive uric acid out of the body which is why it's so good at treating gout. Gout is caused by a build up of uric acid crystals in the joints (cartilage). **Asparagus tea** is another diuretic. So are **water pills**.

List 3:
Immune Stimulants

Suppressor T-Cells suppress the immune response so anything that has the opposite effect (Immunostimulants) should help to counter-act them. Also, of course, a stimulated immune system would aid in the removal of antigens and help to clear the lymph system as well.

Herbs

Cat's Claw, Inner Bark (Uncaria tomentosa) Some of its alkaloids are immune stimulants, and the plant appears to stimulate the activity of T cells. Contains glycosides that exhibit anti-viral and anti-inflammatory activity.

Astragalus Root (Astragalus membranaceus)

The body can develop a tolerance to an adaptogenic herb such as astragalus if it is taken over long stretches of time, (six months). So, for maximum effect, alternate the use of astragalus with other immune-boosting herbs such as Echinacea or Ashwagandha (Withania somnifera), also known as Indian ginseng.

Should not be used if you have a "systemic" disease such as HIV or tuberculosis. This is what some people say and some people say differently so you're going to have to make your own decisions.

Discuss with your health care provider if you are a transplant patient taking immunosuppressive drugs. An immunostimulant could counteract them and lead to organ transplant rejection.

Echinacea Root (Echinacea purpurea)

Cautions

Persons who are allergic to the pollen of other members of the aster family, such as ragweed, may also be allergic to echinacea.

Theoretically, because of potential aggravation of underlying disease state, patients with HIV should not consume echinacea.

A controversy has surrounded the use of echinacea in people infected with HIV. Test tube studies initially showed that echinacea's polysaccharides could increase levels of a substance that might stimulate HIV to spread. However, these results have not been shown to occur when echinacea is taken orally by humans. In fact, one double-blind trial found that *Echinacea angustifolia* root (1 gram three times per day by mouth) greatly increased immune activity against HIV, while placebo had no effect. Further studies are needed to prove the safety of using echinacea in HIV-positive people.

Echinacea stimulates the immune system. It promotes T-cell activation, increases the activity of the immune system and it helps white blood cells to attack germs. These effects may decrease if people take echinacea for more than a few weeks because their immune systems get used to it or develop tolerance to it.

The suggested dosage of echinacea depends on which species and which parts of the plant were used. In general, it should not be used for more than 1-2 weeks at a time.

Echinacea is generally not recommended for people with diseases of the immune system such as HIV, multiple sclerosis, or tuberculosis. The German government recommends against using echinacea if you have these conditions. Some researchers believe that echinacea could actually worsen these immune system problems.

So Why Do People with HIV Use Echinacea?

Many people with HIV have used echinacea because it stimulates the immune system, or for short-term treatment of colds and the flu.

Some doctors believe that it is not a good idea to stimulate the immune system in people who have some type of immune disorder. Increasing the activation of T-cells could give HIV more "target cells" to infect. Other doctors believe that some parts of the immune system are already overactive, causing damage to healthy cells and tissues.

They are also concerned about an animal study showing that echinacea increased levels of tumor necrosis factor alpha (TNF-alpha), a substance produced by the immune system to kill unhealthy cells. High levels of TNF-alpha have been linked to the progression of HIV disease. Of course, if a person's HIV was getting worse then they would have more unhealthy cells, such as cells infected with the virus, especially with fewer immune cells to fight them off and they would need more of this TNF-alpha to fight off such unhealthy cells. The production of this stuff could be the body's natural reaction to try to help itself.

There is no published research to document any dangerous results from the use of echinacea by people with HIV. Unfortunately, as with most herbal products, there is no careful research in people infected with HIV. Some researchers believe that short-term use of echinacea (up to two weeks) to treat colds or flu does not present any serious risks to people with HIV. Also, there are no published studies showing any harmful effects from echinacea. There may be no risk from using echinacea for less than two weeks.

Over Stimulated or Suppressed?

The doctors say that it could be dangerous for people with HIV to take immune stimulants because they think the immune system is already being over stimulated. The old theory is the more viral antigens there are, the more stimulated the immune system is, despite the window of immunogenicity (see vaccines under the supporting evidence section).

However what if the immune system isn't over stimulated

and exhausted; burned out from fighting a losing war against an invincible virus. If the immune system is actually being suppressed then it isn't being over stimulated and an HIV patient could probably take just as many immune stimulants as a normal person.

This is not just a possibility. It is a fact that people with HIV have lower ratios of helper T cells to suppressor T cells, probably caused by a build up of both HIV and self antigens in a partially clogged lymph system so at the very least they should be able to take higher levels of immune stimulants without fear of an overactive immune system or autoimmune disease.

This could also explain why doctors don't have even a shred of evidence that would indicate that people with HIV should not take immune stimulants and why immune stimulants actually seem to help people with HIV. The opposite of suppression is stimulation.

All of these warnings have come from people's theories on the subject. None of these warnings have come from any bad experiences with echinacea so, considering how many people take echinacea, it can be inferred from this that the chances of you having a seriously bad experience would be extremely remote. Remember, all those warnings are entirely without basis. I can say this because they have absolutely no evidence to support them. Some people even say that echinacea isn't an immune stimulant at all. They claim it is an immune tonic and won't cause an over active immune system. Considering that if you take echinacea for more than 1-2 weeks your immune system will become more tolerant of it instead of less they may have a point. If your immune system was going to become overactive it would become overactive to the herb first.

It is also of note that astragalus fits both within the stimulant and adaptogen categories therefore astragalus would definitely be considered an immune tonic because adaptogens make the immune system stronger, even if it also functions as a stimulant. If you can consider astragalus as a tonic then you might also be able to consider echinacea as a tonic.

Bee stings are immune stimulants of a sort and they actually seem to help with the well know autoimmune disease, (arthritis). I cannot explain why, but it may be that immune stimulants do not cause the immune system to become overreactive (except in the case of organ transplants which are foreign bodies). It may be that a little stimulation actually brings the immune system into balance.

If you wanted to take echinacea for longer than 1-2 weeks you would just have to take higher doses for it to still be effective. Personally I don't see a problem with developing a little tolerance. Normally when you develop tolerance to a certain medication we just step up the dosage. This would normally be considered impractical with echinacea because it is normally only used for colds or flu which last only one to two weeks anyway, however while treating a long term illness it may be appropriate.

There is just one problem. Taking the maximum recommended dosage of echinacea is for a short term sprint, like for a cold, but if you take that much echinacea for a long term race it could make your immune system tired and wear it out. Immune stimulants can wear your immune system down, but only if they stress the immune system beyond a certain point. The same thing with how coffee can wear you down, which is also a stimulant. All this means is that you can't take the maximum recommended dosage of echinacea long term or it will wear out your immune system, but just as long as you take a reasonable amount you should be fine. Just remember, a reasonable amount for a long term race is different than a reasonable amount for a sprint.

It really might be best to take echinacea on and off with breaks in between for most people as they recommend, to allow your immune system some rest, but it is true that stimulants can be taken continuously in smaller quantities and for people with suppressed immune systems, they may actually need a little stimulation just to allow their immune systems to be half way awake. Theoretically, their immune systems could get a little stimulation and still get all the rest they need. You might get better results with breaks though. You could also take echinacea with shorter breaks than they recommended, but that is up to you.

Bee stings as immune stimulants

As mentioned before, bee stings are an immune stimulant and they actually seem to help with the well know autoimmune disease (arthritis). Stimulating the immune system in this way seems to help the immune system to reset and reconfigure (or modulate) itself. It could be that immune stimulants may actually decrease the likelihood of getting autoimmune disease.

I heard from my neighbor who is a bee keeper that one doctor just a bit south of where I live purposely takes his patients out just to get stung. Stings do stimulate the immune system, and its benefits to the immune system and arthritis are so great that the patients actually go out there willingly. Arthritis can get bad enough to need that kind of relief.

So that you don't have to go outside you may want to purchase your own pet emperor scorpion to help administer your medication. Now you might say that you wouldn't buy a pet scorpion if your life depended on it, but some people get stung just for arthritis and it could even help your immune system more than immune stimulants from the store so this could be a realistic option. You could have something worse than arthritis. When you buy a scorpion you only have to pay for it once so you could end up saving money, at least in the stimulant category and the treatment outlined in this book would have you buy all kinds of things. Buying bottle after bottle of echinacea could get expensive.

The sting of an emperor scorpion has been described as nothing more than a bad bee sting. You get a lot of venom without a lot of pain, compared to other kinds of scorpions. The more venom you get, the more it stimulates your immune system to work and after a while it won't hurt as much as it did to begin with but just the same it will still stimulate your immune system. You might want to tell your local pet store owner what you're using it for so he can help select the right scorpion for you. Just make sure he's knowledgeable on scorpions. Sometimes small scorpions can hurt more than the big ones. Avoid scorpions with thin pinchers. Thicker pinchers are a sign that they don't need strong venom to subdue their pray. You only need to get stung once a week or so, so it's not too bad. Pain disappears after a couple of hours.

Caution: According to most people, the emperor scorpion sting isn't much worse than a typical bee sting, but if you are allergic to bees don't get a pet scorpion. Some species of scorpions are very dangerous regardless of size so make sure you know what kind of scorpion you're getting. Not everything for sale is always safe. Although the *Pandinus* and *heterometrus* species are considered to be relatively harmless and seldom sting, *Androctonus* and some *Centruroides* species, as well as *Tityus* and *Leiurus*, have caused human deaths.

You may want to buy a young, 4 inch emperor scorpion so that by the time it grows up your body will already be accustomed to the venom. It will also hurt less when you first get it so you'll have time to get used to the idea psychologically. You might not want to buy a really big, 8 inch long, scary looking scorpion and then if you get hurt you might be afraid to get stung a second time, but a small emperor scorpion doesn't hurt any more than a mild bee sting. Some scorpion owners have been known to brag about how often they've been stung so at least to them it's no big deal. This is not too radical of a therapy.

Just be careful of the pinchers. Once an emperor scorpion grows up its pinchers can get strong enough to draw blood. Since the pinchers contain no venom they won't do you any good and there's no point in getting hurt for nothing.

Tarantulas

The bite of a tarantula may be compared with the sting of a bee, though possibly less painful depending on the species. This is only true of pet shop tarantulas. Some tarantulas in the wild can produce extreme discomfort over a period of several days, including spasms, although none of the tarantulas have ever been known to produce human fatalities. The bites of many species are known to be no worse than a wasp sting.

New world tarantulas from North and South America may also flick their legs across their abdomens and throw loose hairs at you, often in little tuffs. These crystalline, barbed hairs can cause variable degrees of skin irritation for a few hours or even days. Don't breathe them in or let them get into your eyes. This may make tarantulas ill suited for this purpose. Old-world tarantulas from Europe, Africa, Asia and Australia do not have these hairs and are more likely to attack when disturbed, but they are often more poisonous.

The bite of a store bought tarantula is only dangerous in that the wound could become infected with bacteria, unless of course you are allergic. Use bactine or antiseptic. As far as I'm concerned, the fact that they can leave a wound with their large fangs disqualifies them from treatment, but that is up to you. The fangs of a large tarantula, such as the Goliath Bird Eater, can inflict painful mechanical injury. Finally, some tarantulas are well known for giving "dry bites," in which they bite, but do not pump venom into the wound.

Allergic to be stings

If you are mildly allergic to bees, a simple cure would be to go out and get stung by just one bee at a time on a routine basis. Be sure to take plenty of antihistamine, like Benadryl for instance.

If you are allergic to peanuts, eat an eighth of a peanut a day. Later you may get up to a quarter or a half a peanut a day. Eventually you should become much more tolerant of what you are allergic to. If you decide to skip the chewing part and just swallow half a peanut with water, if it gets stuck in your throat the inflammation will cut off your breathing. If you eat a peanut, you have to chew the peanut.

According to one of my neighbors, If a person is sensitive to misquote bites, if they get bitten a whole lot, the bites won't bother them anymore.

He also said, one thing about being allergic to bees is that it can go both ways. A person who gets stung once in a while can become less allergic or they can become more allergic. You'd have to get stung at least 4 to 5 times a year to get more tolerant of them. He said bees produce more venom as the summer goes on. They produce the least amount of venom in the spring and by the fall they could be giving out 2 to 3 times more venom so the time you'd want to get stung would be in the spring. He agreed that getting stung once a week (in the spring) would probably cause a persons body to get used to bee stings so they won't be bothered so much. There shouldn't be any significant danger of it going the other way.

My neighbor has studied nursing for 2 years to become a geriatrics CNA (Certified Nursing Assistant). He has an associates' degree and can work at nursing homes and stuff like that. He also learned stuff from the state and the fire department to become a first responder. Besides that he has first hand experience with mosquitoes from when he went to the Korean War.

Mild Arthritis

If you only have mild arthritis and can't stand bees, you could take the maximum recommended dosage of echinacea and astragalus for a brief time to act like a bee sting. Theoretically, it could also cause the immune system to remove any lose microscopic particles of cartilage (cartilage antigens) from around joints that would otherwise trigger an autoimmune response. This might be how stings work. This is only theoretical and I offer no guarantee that it will be effective. You could also take some antihistamine during this time and a little while after to reduce arthritic swelling around joints and to prevent your immune system from attacking your cartilage and worsening the autoimmune condition. Antihistamine is good for allergies even if it's to your own bones. For some reason, antihistamine only seems to act as a potent anti-inflammatory for arthritis when used with a diuretic, possibly because the diuretic carries away uric acid crystals that would otherwise expose cartilage antigens triggering an immune response. Then the antihistamine would keeps what's left of the immune response under control. This combination seems to help both arthritis and gout induced arthritis. Only an antihistamine will do this. Anti-inflammatories will not.

Licorice is an anti-inflammatory suggested for rheumatoid arthritis, although aspirin (which comes from willow bark) might be better. This may also be useful for chronically inflamed lymph nodes. Wintergreen has aspirin like properties and may be used to reduce joint and muscle inflammation. Other things for inflammation include wild yam and black cohosh. Don't take either of these while pregnant. Ibuprofen is another anti-inflammatory that seems to help arthritis.

Celery seed is especially effective against gout and gout induced arthritis. You see in gout, uric acid crystals build up in the joints, especially in the far extremities of the body, like the big toe, where circulation is sluggish. Where circulation is slow, uric acid falls out of solution and precipitates into crystals. Washing your hands a lot in cold water can also cause uric acid to fall out of solution due to the temperature change. Cold causes the blood vessels to constrict and decrease circulation, even if it's just on the surface of the skin. These needle shaped crystals then stab your cartilage, causing inflammation and exposing cartilage antigens to your immune system. This can stimulate the autoimmune disease, rheumatoid arthritis and repeated gout attacks can damage bone.

If you buy some cayenne powder and put it into empty gelatin capsules, this can be used to increase circulation even to the point of simulating a mild fever. Cayenne dilates blood vessels. You may want to take some milk and cereal or ice cream with it to protect your stomach.

Celery seed is a diuretic and it can be used in getting rid of these crystals. When they thought my uncle had gout, the doctor prescribed a diuretic. Diet can also be adjusted for gout. Boiled burdock root has been used for arthritis, gout, lung disease, and as a mild laxative, "a diuretic," and as a perspiration inducer. Along with nettle, which increases circulation, it has been used against rheumatism and gout. Since celery seed is used in getting rid of these crystals and lymphagogues aren't, it may be even more effective than lymphagogues for removing at least certain wastes. However, uric acid is also found in lymph fluid, so a lymphagogue used in combination with a diuretic should work better than a diuretic alone.

Stimulants - Tree Extracts, Herbs, Flowers, Mushrooms and Such

Many people are familiar with immune supplements like astragalus, echinacea, arabinogalactan, goldenseal (anti-viral/ anti-bacterial properties) and phytosterol's like beta-sitosterol (Th1, Th2 balance). Many of these are stimulants and push parts of the immune system to expand or go faster. These and others can be found singularly or in combinations. Together, they can be quite effective for a short while. Responsible manufacturers will caution that stimulants are for short-term use (2 weeks perhaps).

Immune System Stimulation Has a Limited Effect

One of the reasons short-term use (as opposed to long term use) of stimulants is recommended is because over stimulation of the immune system can lead to immune system exhaustion. Everyone's immune system, according to Dr. Stoff, functions from a baseline level. That level could be high (not many of us), very low (common) or anywhere in between. In relationship to Natural Killer cell activity, stimulation will cause an initial rise in NK activity but after a short period of time the stimulation will diminish and the NK activity will return to baseline, or below. He also says that stimulation does not affect the immune system as a whole.

Drugs

There are a number of prescription drugs for stimulating the immune system, but for prescriptions of any kind consult your doctor. Prescription drugs can be dangerous and should only be prescribed by a trained medical professional on an individual basis.

List 4:
Immune Modulators

Immune System stimulants work entirely differently than does an Immune Modulator. Stimulants increase the activity of all kinds of elements of the Immune System, indiscriminately. Immune Modulators enable the body to increase or decrease the activity of each element of the Immune System as appropriate to the body's needs in any given situation. It brings an underactive immune system up and brings an overactive immune system down.

Instead of having either a "Weak" Immune System or an "Overactive" one, some of us may actually have an "Impaired" Immune System. This is indicated by the fact that someone may have a Common Cold, which is associated with a "Weak" Immune System, and at the same time have Asthma, which is considered an Auto-Immune Disorder. Auto-Immune Disorders are thought to be the result of an "overactive" Immune System attacking healthy body tissue. An Immune System Modulator is capable of assisting the body to address both conditions at the same time.

Chronic fatigue syndrome: Also as you might remember from the supporting evidence section of this book, people with chronic fatigue syndrome have been found to have both high and low ratios of helper T cells to suppressor T cells. This could be a sign of a poorly regulated immune system so you'd think that an Immune modulator would be all that they would need, however...

Chronic fatigue syndrome usually starts out suddenly, accompanied by a flu-like illness. Also the patient may have one of several viruses that stays with them for the rest of their life which is like HIV, although it is not fatal. In fact another name for chronic fatigue syndrome is Post-Viral Fatigue Syndrome (PVFS). A few of these viruses are also retroviruses, again like HIV and as you might remember from the supporting evidence section, some retroviruses may manipulate regulatory T cells into suppressing the immune system of the host. Some parasites may also do this (as in elephantiasis). It is possible that just about anything can, hence one of chronic fatigue syndrome's other names: Post-infectious fatigue syndrome (PIFS). They even have a post Lyme disease syndrome called post-Lyme syndrome where the Lyme disease bacteria stays with the patient for years.

Chronic fatigue also makes you more prone to cancer it is thought because of your weakened immune system so it is also known as chronic fatigue immune dysfunction syndrome (CFIDS). Full recovery from chronic fatigue occurs in only 5-10% of cases. Most people don't recover from AIDs or tuberculosis either.

It seems the most effective treatment we have for chronic fatigue is pacing back and forth, probably because it moves the lymph fluid.

So people with chronic fatigue syndrome may also benefit from the same treatments used for cancer and HIV mentioned in this book. However, I doubt that immune modulators would be enough by themselves.

Transfer Factor Plus Advanced Formula

Independent lab tests have proven that Transfer Factor Plus Advanced Formula increases the Natural Killer (NK) cell activity by 437%. This NK function is a major component of your immune system that destroys (lyses) virus-infected cells and tumor cells. Echinacea only increased this function by 43%. In addition Echinacea and most other herbs are immune stimulants. They can't be taken continuously or they will wear out your immune system. Transfer Factor Plus Advanced is an immune modulator. It only activates when a virus or germ of some kind is present. It provides constant protection, and can be taken every day without causing any problems.

Transfer Factor Plus Advanced Formula has been proven in independent lab studies to increase the activity of the Natural Killer cells by 248% above normal. The level or activity of NK cells in chronic fatigue syndrome, cancer, and chronic viral infections is usually low.

Transfer Factor Plus Advanced Formula from 4Life™ Research is a scientifically advanced formulation of transfer factors from two different sources, plus additional all natural ingredients. The sources are bovine colostrum and chicken egg yolks. This combination of transfer factors increases the Natural Killer cell activity by 437%.

Warning: Do not use this product if you have an organ transplant or during pregnancy.

Ai/E10

There are no side effects other than those associated with healing. It's not colostrum or dairy. Those with dairy intolerance need not be concerned. It's safe to use with autoimmune diseases. It's safe for babies. It's safe for your dog. Your body sees the immune factors in Ai/E10 extract as its own. These factors are biologically engineered but entirely natural. There's no difference between the immune factors in Ai/E10 extract and those found in your body.

Whether your immune system is underactive or overactive, Ai/E10 extract can help bring your immune system into balance by restoring communication pathways, regulating immune function, increasing NK cell activity and acting as a general all-around immune regulator to help with the utilization of nutrients.

It activates NK cells and total immune response including T-suppressor cells. It also influences the T helper cell profile and has been recognized to support cytokine pathways utilized by the body in cell to cell communication. Ai/E10 is also called Antigen Infused Dialyzable Bovine Colostrum/Whey Extract (AIDBCWE).

Thymus Extracts

Thymus extracts may provide a solution to chronic viral infection and low immune function. Thymus extract has been shown to normalize the ratio of T helper cells to suppressor cells, whether the ratio is low (as in AIDS and cancer) or high (as in allergies or rheumatoid arthritis).

Adaptogens

Adaptogens are often combined for a more potent synergistic effect. An example is astragalus and ligustrum; the combination is more effective than either plant used alone.

<u>**Astragalus**</u> *(Astragalus membranaceus)*

Actions: Immune stimulant; adaptogenic; vasodilator, improves circulation; anti-viral. **Uses:** Tonic and endurance remedy; immune stimulant (not an acute remedy, like echinacea, but for long-term use to improve immune function); and night sweats.

One of the premier tonic herbs of China; astragalus builds energy and helps warm up the body. It is one of the most important double-direction immune modulating herbs in the world.

Astragalus membranaceus root has a centuries-long history of use, in China. Today, we know that this herb is able to foster normal immune response in cancer and AIDS patients, to correct T-cell deficiency, and to promote antiviral action. Combined with ligustrum, it is available in extract and capsule form. These two herbs can also be bought whole, then crushed, and then simmered in a small amount of water for several hours. The Chinese prepare herbs in this way and consume them daily.

Often used in conjunction with astragalus and ligustrum is the ganoderma, or reishi mushroom. This is a general energy stimulant, digestive aid, and cancer-fighter. Reishi mushroom has long been used in the Orient to help those recovering from chronic illness, especially general weakness.

Astragalus has many potential applications and few, if any, side effects. Astragalus has no known harmful side effects, but taking large concentrated amounts for a prolonged period, in the form of extracts or capsules may cause abdominal and chest tension in some people.

Active Constituents: The interpene glycosides, saponins, the total astragaloside fraction of astragalus (trademarked as TA-70), is an extremely potent immune modulator capable of building the immune response while suppressing excessive immune activity as occurs in autoimmune conditions (i.e. allergies and arthritis) and is an extremely potent antioxidant.

Supreme Protector

Supreme Protector is an ultimate Chinese protective formulation. It is composed of the three kings of defense in Chinese Herbalism: Reishi, Astragalus and **Cordyceps.** All protect the body, mind and spirit in various ways. Each is a potent immune modulator and all have powerful anti-stress activity. They all have antioxidant action, and are highly adaptogenic.

Protector 2000 is as potent an immune system protector as you can find. It contains the three strongest immune modulators known to Chinese herbalism, which is saying a lot. **Agaricus mushroom** is now known to be the most potent immune modulator in the world. **Reishi spores** are 7 times more potent as an immune system modulator than Reishi mushroom extract (and Reishi mushrooms are one of the strongest immune modulators in the world). **Lycium polysaccharides** have been demonstrated to have very potent immune potentiating action. This formula will build your immune system.

Prime One -

Stress and not getting enough rest could very well be degrading your health. When you are overworked, things begin to break down and without the needed time for recuperation your body cannot repair itself. Your internal organs and insides actually do get smaller. It's like starvation with exercise. Your body doesn't just need food. It needs time to utilize it. If your cells aren't healthy, then they can't perform their functions properly and whatever they are a part of can't be healthy. That's why stress wears you down. Adaptogens help your body to build itself up.

Adaptogens support the built in capacities of the body's own self regulatory defense systems. They release your own innate energy, vitality and strength to help you to be at your best. They cause the body to respond to stress as though it were exercise. One adaptogen may do this for your muscles, another for your immune system.

Too many immune stimulants can stress the immune system, but now all that stress could be converted into exercise. Immune stimulants could be used to exercise the immune system and build it up, theoretically. If your immune system is being suppressed, it probably wouldn't get much exercise otherwise and probably wouldn't get much stronger from adaptogens alone. Where would the exercise come from to adapt to without stimulants?

At the Olympic Games the soviet team dominated the World Ice Hockey championships up till 1983, winning the gold an amazing 15 times over a 20-year period. They were not using steroids or drugs. They never even had a single drug violation. They were using an incredible all-natural secret blend of adaptogens.

Adaptogens work better together and Prime One contains the most incredible formulation of adaptogens ever conceived. It contains 7 adaptogens and the history of its development is the most fascinating I have ever encountered.

Now considered the number one product for stress relief in the world, the formula now used in "Prime One" was adaptogenically developed and tested for 45 years by Dr. Israel I. Brekhman and a team of Russian scientists in the former Soviet Union at an estimated cost of over 1 Billion dollars. Since then 1,200 scientists in more than 3,000 clinical studies have substantiated the effectiveness of the formula now used in Prime One on stress relief in tens of thousands of Russian citizens. Prime One has even been tested for use by children.

The 7 adaptogens include: Eleutherococcus senticosus- king of adaptogens, counteracts stress and increases endurance, **Glycyrrhiza uralensis-** Supports immunity, **Schizandra chinesis-** combats fatigue, **Rhaponticum carthamoides-** enhances your muscles and improves circulation, **Aralia mandshurica-** Enhances mental acuity, **Crataegus oxycantha-** Promotes cardiac stability, **Rhodiola rosea-** improves physical and mental performance.

This once protected secret formula was created by the Russian Academy of Sciences to give Olympic athletes, cosmonauts, KGB agents, military leaders and others an unstoppable edge over the rest of the world. During the cold war, 1,200 of the Soviet Union's most accomplished scientists were ordered to develop this performance-enhancing formula to prove the superiority of the country's elite and its communist system to the world. Olympic athletes, cosmonauts, KGB agents, military leaders, and others would be "under orders" to take this formula every morning.

For twenty years in the former Soviet Union, Dr. Brekhman researched and used natural nutritional supplements for elite athletes. These secrets gave the Soviet Olympic teams a key competitive advantage, especially in enhancing performance and restoration, which is also what you need if you're sick. It was not until The Collapse of The Soviet Union in 1991 that their governments' secret formula was discovered.

In its development there were some requirements that the formula had to meet. It must:

- be 100% natural, after athletes were banned from using steroids and performance enhancing drugs
- not interact with any medications
- be 100% non-toxic
- instantly create a long-idling surge of energy and improve stamina

- stimulate the body's immune system
- promote peak performance in every way and shorten recovery time

Supercharges Immunity Adaptogens are powerful immune modulators, helping you build resistance to infectious disease and prevent auto immune reactions. They help maintain the health and integrity of your cells and have even been shown to have anti-cancer effects.

Things like "Prime One" that will boost your energy can be quite helpful regardless of their direct impact on immune function. Because they make it easier for you to exercise you will move more and this will help to move the lymph system. If you are more active, then you can be more proactive in taking care of yourself.

Coffee will give you energy by allowing you to overexert yourself. This is also what fear does. Don't use stimulants. Only use things that give you energy by making you stronger. A nap will do this.

Excessive use of nervous stimulants stresses the nervous system. Coffee contains caffeine, which is a central nervous stimulant. The use of stimulants on a long term basis is to be avoided, since they will rapidly deplete the body's energy reserves and lead to exhaustion.

List 5: Unburdening the immune system

We all have germs growing both on us and in us. These germs are not normally considered bad germs because our immune systems keep them in check, however with an impaired immune system even relatively harmless germs can grow to excessively large proportions and under these conditions just about anything that can grow on or inside of you will. This includes bacteria, fungi, yeast, and just about anything else. An AIDS patient can be like an old tree just covered in moss, fungi, and mold.

This can put quite a burden on your immune system, or lymph system, as well as cause a toxic build up of germ excretions, causing mild poisoning. There might not even be any symptoms except for tiredness, possibly aches and pains, and a general feeling of unhealthiness.

The fact that there are only mild symptoms with this many bacteria in the body indicates that it might not be because the immune system has been wiped out, but because after the bacteria have infected a person and spread their antigens everywhere in a lymph system that is already backed up, it could cause tolerance for the bacteria. AIDs patients are sickly already so they would ordinarily have more bacteria in their systems. Here, bacteria would be spreading high levels of antigens around in a system that's already clogged. The level of antigens would be high because a clogged lymph system can't get rid of them.

This is actually good news. It means that if the damaged

immune system is just extremely tolerant rather than being almost completely wiped out then there's more of the immune system left than we thought and we could restore more of the immune system than we originally thought possible.

In order to help the immune system to recuperate from its weakened state it might be a good idea to get rid of all the secondary infections and other things that it has to deal with that burden it down. In fact it's not actually the AIDS virus that kills an AIDS patient, but all of these secondary infections.

Goldenseal

Active ingredients: berberine and hydrastine alkaloids. Both exhibit strong antibacterial and even anti-viral effects. Berberine has been shown to kill a variety of germs and parasites such as yeast infections, tapeworms and giardia. Many researchers believe that it may also be capable of activating white blood cells. Thus, goldenseal is used as an all-around disinfectant, both externally and internally. However it is believed to exhibit only a localized effect in the gastrointestinal track as its alkaloids, especially berberine, are not well absorbed into the bloodstream, limiting any reaching antibiotic effects.

Main use: Colds and flu, upper respiratory infections, and chronic fatigue syndrome. Goldenseal tea is taken for stomachaches. It is one of the most effective herbal remedies for inflammation of the mucous membranes and strongly stimulates the secretion of bile (like the coffee enema). It is also said to enhance the potency of other herbs.

CAUTION: Do not use for more than 10 days consecutively without giving several weeks off in between, as there is a property that tends to build up in the liver and causes the liver to become toxic over long term use.

Colloidal silver

Colloidal Silver is a non-toxic anti-microbial, viricide, bactericide, fungicide and disinfectant to remedy sore throats, colds, thrush, acne, rashes, septic wounds and numerous other ailments. From the article, "Silver, Our Mightiest Germ Fighter," in Science Digest, March, 1978: "As an antibiotic, colloidal silver kills over 650 disease causing organisms, and resistant strains fail to develop.

Silver functions as a catalyst to disable the enzymes that many bacteria, fungi, and viruses use for their metabolism. Unlike many antibiotics, silver helps kill only the bacteria that are anaerobic. Friendly bacteria in the digestive tract and in other areas of the body that are aerobic are not affected.

Prior to 1938, colloidal silver was widely used by physicians as a mainstream antibiotic. It was produced by pharmaceutical companies under various names, including Protargol. But the electro-colloidal production process was costly and the pharmaceutical industry developed fast-acting, less-expensive sulfa drugs and penicillin. ~Wikipedia

Colloidal silver antibacterial liquid has been sprayed on Hong Kong subways as a public health measure. From NaturalNews: Subway and train stations in London and other parts of the UK are considering using a powerful, non-toxic colloidal silver disinfectant spray to help fend off the spread of the flu virus this winter after Hong Kong subways recently announced its use of the spray.

Silver is also used by the Soviets to sterilize recycled water aboard the Mir Space Station. Silver filters can be found in the water fountains of every airliner and spacecraft to guarantee germ-free water. Silver is even being used to replace chlorine in swimming pools, because it does not sting the eyes and offers great germicidal action.

If you are a doctor and are not entirely familiar with colloidal silver, it's because pharmaceutical companies no longer advertize it as they once did, but when it comes to peoples' health, sometimes you've got to do your own research.

Considerations

Colloidal Silver is non-toxic, but if you drink too much of it at a time, it is theoretically possible that it could kill too many bad germs all at once. Toxins stored in the germs would be released into your system and your body could get overwhelmed with trying to get rid of all of the dead germ corpses and fluids. It is possible to feel a little sick because, if you have HIV or an impaired immune system, you could end up poisoning yourself. Many of these toxins and waste materials would have to be removed through the lymph system so be sure to take something to help the lymph fluid to flow better. If it gets plugged up the toxins will stay in your system longer so be sure to drink plenty of liquids at this time so you can pee it all out. Keep your liver and kidneys in mind. They may have to deal with a large volume of waste, but only if you take an unusually large volume of colloidal silver.

Don't worry about taking too much of it. If you drank a large volume of colloidal silver, the worst that could theoretically happen is that you might feel a little sick or polluted temporarily. Just follow the directions on the bottle. You'll be fine.

Some people may fear that too much colloidal silver could kill off friendly bacteria in the intestines. Just to prove that this is not so, a man named Mark Metcalf of Los Angeles, California made a 16 ounce solution of well over 250 parts per million colloidal silver and drank it. He repeated this procedure every day for 4 days in a row. He said "I easily drank the equivalent of 50 sixteen-once glasses of 5 PPM colloidal silver every day!" This is the equivalent of 25 16-once glasses of 10 PPM or 8 and a third 16-once glasses of 30 PPM. He did not eat yogurt, acidophilus, or compensate for friendly bacteria in any way. He said "The only side effect was that I just seemed to feel better." This comes to you from the 1998 volume 2 - number 1 issue of Exotic Research Report. The magazine is now known as Extraordinary Technology produced by Tesla-Tech.

Colloidal silver is entirely non-toxic and the above theory of bacterial poisoning would only apply to some rare individuals, if the theory is even correct.

If you decide to make your own colloidal silver at home, you actually could make an entire gallon of colloidal silver. The instructions on a bottle of store bought colloidal silver are for the common cold and to save money so it makes since that you would want a little more silver than that for a more advanced illness.

You can find instructions on the internet for how to make your own colloidal silver using only a battery or a transformer (AC or DC), two pieces of pure silver metal and a glass of water. It involves a sort of electroplating method, but if your water has a lot of nitrate in it, silver nitrate building up in your skin could cause your skin to turn blue. This harmless and infrequent cosmetic condition is known as argyria. I've heard that some people with argyria still take colloidal silver just because it makes them feel better.

Even though to the best of my knowledge, there is no record of anyone contracting argyria from colloidal silver made by the electrolytic method, you can avoid this problem by using only pure water, perhaps from a bottled (bottled water). Use only pure silver, also known as fine silver. Do not use a silver-copper alloy or you'll be drinking copper. Sterling silver contains nearly 8% copper.

Colloidal silver spray

If you have tuberculosis you could put colloidal silver in a spray bottle and spray it into your lungs as you inhale. It should be a very fine mist. Make sure it's only colloidal silver. Some types of colloidal silver are watered down (as in 10 parts per million compared to 30 parts per million) and you don't want to be spraying water into your lungs. Actually, the water should be absorbed into your tissues so it might not hurt anything. As it turns out they already make spray bottles of colloidal silver specifically for this purpose with instructions right on the bottle! You could also try swallowing some colloidal silver down the wrong tube, but that might get uncomfortable.

HIV is not fatal for everyone and some people have gotten

better before this book was even written. HIV does not have a 100% mortality rate, so don't give up hope. Believe in yourself. The progression of a disease is not up to the germ. Its fate is determined by your actions.

A Simple Basic Test Run [Just to try it out]

This probably won't cure you. It's just to see if it will make you feel any better or not. Then if it looks to you like this sort of treatment will help you to recover, you could pursue the matter further. That's what test runs are for. For the most affordable, most available, and quickest and easiest to obtain remedy I can think of, while still maintaining a pretty decent level of quality try:

Red Clover Stillingia *Lymphagogue or lymph thinner* From "Herb Pharm" 1 fluid once, liquid herbal extract. Contains pokeweed root. My grandmother had breast cancer and the doctors had to surgically remove one of her breasts. Her lymph fluid in her arm was bothering her. 55 drops twice a day made it go away. 40 drops twice a day had no effect at all.

This is just temporary. After taking pokeweed for a while you'll probably have to switch to something else because pokeweed has a tendency to build up in the liver. Lymphagogue, Iris versicolor has been used as a blood purifier and to treat diseases of the liver. Alternate your lymphagogues for maximum effect.

Note: Red Clover Stillingia_compound contains only small amounts of pokeweed among many other herbs. The active ingredient that thins lymph fluid is primarily Stillingia and there is no warning label on the bottle about this sort of thing so actually it is pretty safe.

<u>**A Diuretic:**</u> Lymphagogues should be taken with **celery seed**. Celery seed is a *diuretic* and together they could really help to clean out the body. The idea is, the lymph thinner makes the lymph system have more fluid and then the diuretic gets rid of it and all the wastes there in. Lymphagogues make the lymph more watery, but celery seed makes it move. Together they create a flow through your body. Of course, celery seed won't work alone because the lymph just isn't watery enough.

A diuretic makes you pee more often. If you can't see any difference in how many times a day you have to go to the bathroom, just take a little more celery seed.

Warning: People who take diuretics to lose weight (water weight) may end up with a potassium deficiency. They may also pee out a lot of their nutrition. Too many water pills can also affect the heart.

I'm just concerned about one thing with diuretics. It's easy to get dehydrated with diuretics so it's easy for your lymph fluid to get dehydrated. Dehydrated lymph fluid won't flow properly. You don't want your diuretic to defeat the purpose of your lymphagogue. Drink plenty of Ice tea, lemonade or punch. It doesn't have to be pure water because once it gets to your stomach and mixes with whatever you've eaten; it won't be pure water anyway. The body absorbs a lot of water through the intestines and once it gets there, it won't be pure water anymore. If your water tastes good and you keep it readily available you might drink more of it. Soda can be hard on the kidneys though. Keep a pitcher next to you. You might not bother to fill up your glass if your pitcher is far away.

Colloidal Silver *antibiotic* from "Source Naturals": 30 parts per million. It comes in 2 fluid once bottles.

All Thymus *modulator* from "Natural Sources": All Thymus is a raw thymus glandular concentrate with synergistic complex.

Reishi mushroom Or one of the other mushrooms. They're all based on polysaccharides so they all fulfill sort of the same function.

Echinacea and Astragalus Something from both the *stimulant* and *adaptogen* categories. This is necessary to provide a kick start to the treatment. It gets things going and puts things in motion. You might not see much without it. In fact if you took just these two with a diuretic and took the maximum recommended dosage of the red clover Stillingia along with a bit of walking to move your lymph fluid, you should be able to get better results and save money on your test run.

Test run:

1. Lymph thinner / Stillingia
2. Diuretic / celery seed
3. Immune stimulant / Echinacea
4. Adaptogen / Astragalus

+ Pacing / exercise

CHAPTER 4

The Real Treatment

You might want to specialize in these 4 categories (adaptogens, immune stimulants, lymph thinners, and a diuretic). In fact if you took just twice the maximum recommended dosages of these 4 items, it might be enough to theoretically reverse the progression of HIV for a short time, but since that would not be practical you could take the maximum recommended dosages of 2 or 3 different items from each of the first 3 categories. This way you would never have to take more than the maximum recommended dosage of any one item.

No matter how many items you take from different categories, if you are not taking something to thin you lymph fluid you are not getting the real treatment. Exercise alone will not move a congested lymph system properly. Also if you took 2 or 3 different things to thin your lymph fluid it would be like taking 2 or 3 times the dosage of just one item alone.

Taking the maximum recommended dosages from the stimulant, adaptogen, and lymph thinner categories, along with a diuretic, I consider to be the purified and refined treatment.

An immune stimulant, an adaptogen, and something to thin the lymph fluid along with a diuretic to clear out the wastes is all that's necessary to provide the mechanism at the heart of the treatment discussed in this book.

This is a bare bones treatment and even though it does help to specialize in these 4 areas you can also take things from other categories to help strengthen your immune system such as immune modulators and mushrooms which also have immune stimulating effects. I'm guessing that most people might decide to take things from other categories. Just don't get distracted with variety ahead of effectiveness.

With this treatment, you do have to put forth some effort and it is mildly expensive. Just about anything that actually works is expensive. It wouldn't be like you could just drive down to the health food store and pick up some pills like there's nothing to it. You have to take a lot of things and some high quality things as well.

Don't think that it's unusual for doctors to recommend such high levels of medication. Doctors routinely prescribe chemo therapy (or chemical therapy) where they give their patients chemicals and drugs in such high levels that it makes their hair fall out! It takes a lot. This is serious.

Taking antibiotics like golden root and colloidal silver is not part of the real treatment although if you have an impaired immune system (HIV) they can help. The real treatment is your immune system. Antibiotics have no direct roll in breaking the tolerance so they are in their own separate classification. Also if you have cancer and you do not have anything else wrong with you, antibiotics may be nearly useless.

I have no problem with the idea of you taking slightly less than a medium dose of echinacea long term without breaks. According to Wikipedia; "the safety of echinacea under long term use is unknown," therefore no one can say that it is dangerous and if it was I think we would know by now. As long as you do not stimulate your immune system beyond a certain point, echinacea will not wear down your immune system. However, if you take echinacea continuously, your immune system may become more tolerant of echinacea over time up to a point. It will still stimulate your immune system, but it just won't work as well as it did at first.

Even a small amount of immune stimulation is many times stronger than none at all. A little under a medium dose of echinacea long term should be fine even once your immune system has become fairly tolerant of it just as long as you are taking plenty of other things with it to help strengthen your immune system. However, the maximum recommended dosage of echinacea is for short term spurts like with a cold and taking that high of a dosage in a long term race without breaks could wear out you immune system. Short term spurts off and on are recommended and that's what most people do.

You must take exercise with this treatment. It is required that you pace back and forth frequently throughout the day or at least go for a walk once a day. Thinning the lymph fluid won't do any good if it's not moving. Taking exercise is just like taking any of the other pills. Pacing is currently the most effective single treatment we have for chronic fatigue syndrome. If you are not taking exercise, you are not on the treatment.

What Comes First?

If you have something as bad as HIV, you could take echinacea with breaks and scorpion stings during those breaks. Don't worry about it wearing out your immune system. It's a different kind of stimulant.

Remember, the key to this treatment is just to take everything you can and as much as possible; first and foremost from the (1st) stimulant and (2^{d}) lymph thinner categories, then (3^{d}) diuretics and (4th) adaptogens, and then (5th) immune modulators and mushrooms.

I put immune stimulants in first place because they are the only category known to fight off arthritis. None of the other categories are known to do that (arthritis is not gout). Also, the opposite of suppression is stimulation. If you don't plan on getting "stung" at least once a week, even with echinacea, then lymph thinners and diuretics take first place. They tried using immune modulators against chronic fatigue syndrome with only poor results.

Because Transfer Factor Plus (*modulator*) works so well, perhaps it should be bumped up a level of importance or two. It's difficult to gauge these things because they have different levels of strength.

Gauging Effectiveness

If you have HIV and you come down with flu-like symptoms and feel absolutely terrible, that might just be your immune system kicking in. It could be a sign that your immune system is finally responding to the virus. Of course this would mean a drastic and sudden drop in the level of tolerance so this probably wouldn't happen. More likely you'd just feel like you were getting a little healthier. The tolerance would come down slowly and the number of viruses would slowly come down with it.

What to Use

All of the ingredients mentioned in the test run could easily be replaced by others. For example colloidal silver could easily be replaced with sodium chlorite [NaClO2]. When mixed with vinegar it produces chlorine dioxide which, in 1999, the American Society of Analytical Chemists stated was the most powerful pathogen killer known to man. Mix 20 drops with 3 teaspoons of vinegar, close lid of very small bottle, wait 3 minutes, then drink. Available at [Websites:] http://www.health4allinfo.ca and http://www.miraclemineral.org. Brand name: **Miracle mineral solution.**

If you want to kick it up a notch, a much more effective and much more expensive treatment would be **"Transfer Factor Plus"** to replace the "all thymus," **Prime One** to make you strong all over, and **cleavers or New Jersey tea**. Because they are non-toxic you could take far more of them than you could pokeweed or Iris versicolor (poison flag).

CHAPTER 5

What You Can do to Help Yourself

If you need to lose some weight and exercise or if you need treatment or something like that, it does not have to be an act of self mutilation, but it won't work if you don't treat it like it's your job either. If you miss a couple days of work in a row you'll get fired and the same thing here. Just doing a light but reasonable amount of work, like how you would do your homework, will do. Exercise can be light just as long as it's consistent. The main reason why so many diets fail is because diets only work when you're on them. You've got to take it seriously.

You can't put forth much effort without motivation. If you need motivation then you would need a goal or something to think about. If you think about what you want then it will help you to get there. Even if it's hard you may find a way to get there anyway. Do not accept the way your life is now. Instead, think about how you want things to be. You need to daydream about doing a really good job and making things a whole lot better. Then you'll have the same kind of desire that I have.

Later you may have to decide which course of action you should take in your treatment even if you are not qualified to do so. I was not really qualified to make progress in both the fields of cancer and AIDS, but I did. Now, you must decide what to study, which treatment to take and which treatment you cannot afford.

You may also be able help your friends and neighbors. If you know anyone with cancer, HIV, tuberculosis, elephantiasis, chronic fatigue syndrome, or anyone on chemo-therapy bring this to their attention and try to help them. It is possible to use my method without a prescription, so it should be quite safe and it would probably make things much easier on the patient than whatever ailments they may be going through now. Here are some various things you might want to look up on the internet:

- Co-stimulation & antigen presenting cells
- Suppressor T cells and how they suppress the immune response. *See also* Regulatory T Cells
- (Immuno-regulatory agents) such as drugs and herbs that can stimulate the production of antigen presenting cells
- How to drain the lymph system of toxins. ~This is the most important thing

Don't stop reading now because this book isn't over yet, as the ending lies with you.

Author Jason Mc Kenna

Sources:

Organized by book chapter

The Theory

"How HIV Causes AIDS, NIAID Facts Sheet" as seen in chapter 1 (The Theory): National Institute of Allergy and Infectious Diseases, National Institutes of Health, U.S. Department of Health and Human Services. Website: http://www.niaid.nih.gov/factsheets/howhiv.htm Telephone Toll-Free: 866-284-4107 Fax: 301-402-3573 U.S. Mail NIAID Office of Communications and Government Relations 6610 Rockledge Drive, MSC 6612 Bethesda, MD 20892-6612 USA. This is the source for the sections entitled "Slow Viruses" and "Early Events in HIV Infection" located at the beginning of this book.

Immunological tolerance Kimball's Biology Pages: http://users.rcn.com/jkimball.ma.ultranet/BiologyPages/T/Tolerance.html

Regulatory T cells, same place, different web page: http://users.rcn.com/jkimball.ma.ultranet/BiologyPages/T/Treg.html

Regulatory T cells (also known as **suppressor T Cells**) Wikipedia, the free encyclopedia Web Page: http://en.wikipedia.org/wiki/Regulatory_T_cells

The Solution

The Coffee Enema - A Liver Cleanser "S.A. Wilsons Therapy Blend Coffee" web site: http://www.sawilsons.com/liver.htm Based upon Dr. Gerson's work. More information is available in his book: ***A Cancer Therapy, Results of Fifty Cases.*** Mail: s.a. Wilson's 2891 Regional Road 20 Bowmanville, Ontario Canada L1C 3K6 Phone: 905-263-2344 or 1-866-266-4066 Fax: 905-263-4764 E-mail: scott@sawilsons.com <mailto:scott@sawilsons.com>

Manual lymphatic drainage (MLD) Cancerbackup, the UK's leading cancer information charity. Learn about MLD, Simple lymphatic drainage (self massage), and Deep breathing exercises. Web Site: http://www.cancerbackup.org.uk/Home Free phone Helpline: 0808 -800 -1234

Lymph Drainage Therapy, The latest techniques for proven success. The International Alliance of Healthcare Educators. web site: http://www.iahe.com/html/therapies/ldt.jsp IAHE General Contact Info: 11211 Prosperity Farms Rd. D-325 Palm Beach Gardens, FL 34410-3487 USA Phone: 561-622-4334 Toll-Free: 800-311-9204 Fax: 561-622-4771 E-mail: iahe@iahe.com <mailto:iahe@iahe.com>

The Lymphatic Center™ A Natural Healthcare & Education Center. Web site: http://www.merc-buyers.com/about_lymphatics.htm Internet and phone consultations available.

Hours by Appointment. Carol Ann Santella, C.L.,HC Phone: (412) -681 -1105 Office location: Pittsburgh, Pa USA

Health Wake-Up Merger -Promoting a healthy life style. Web site: http://www.healthwakeup.co.za/contact us.htm Tel: +27 11 791 4008 Fax: +27 11 791 3833 Unit 11, c/r Susan & Langwa Sts, Strijdom Park, Randburg, 2162 P O Box 1412, Ferndale, 2160 Gauteng, South Africa (za) They mentioned that wheat and dairy products can easily clog the lymphatic system.

Lymphstar Pro and a significant amount of data on the lymphatic system comes to you from: "Accelerated-Wellness" -Complementing Main Stream Medicine. http://www.accelerated-wellness.com/lymph-drainage.htm Telephone: 317-865-0889 General Information: therapist@accelerated-wellness.com <mailto:therapist@accelerated-wellness.com> Postal address: 925 E. Southport Rd., Indianapolis, IN 46227

Flexitouch® The Flexitouch consists of inflating and deflating garments that can give the patient a manual lymphatic drainage massage. The Flexitouch® Lymphedema System can only be prescribed by a physician. "Tactile Systems Technology, Inc." http://www.tactilesystems.com/html/reimbursement.html For Customer Service Call: 866-4 Flexitouch. That's 866-435-3948

"**The Reynolds Office of Health and Nutrition**" Serving the Natural Health Community since 1985. Sue Reynolds, Master Herbalist The Reynolds Office of Health and Nutrition P.O. Box 591, Goleta, CA 93116 http://www.reynoldsoffice.com/3171-7.htm Call or Write Us for More Information Phone: 805-692-6912 Email:Herbalist@ReynoldsOffice.com <mailto:Herbalist@ReynoldsOffice.com&subject=Information Request - contact (reynoldsoffice.com)>

Gerald M. Lemole, M.D. talks about heart transplant surgery cutting the lymphatics and the associated risk of atherosclerosis, or blockage of the arteries, in monkeys, but mostly he just talks a lot about lymph fluid, diet, and care. From the desk of Clarence Bass of "Ripped Enterprises." Web site: http://cbass.com/lymph.htm Contact Information: Telephone 505-266-5858 (M-F, 8-5 Mountain time) FAX 505-266-9123 International fax: 001-505-266-9123 Note: Check your local phone book for faxing instructions. Postal address P.O. Box 51236, Albuquerque, New Mexico 87181-1236 U.S.A. E-mail General Information: cncbass@aol.com (e-mail <mailto:cncbass@aol.com>) Don't send attachments or photos. Company policy prohibits the downloading of either of them. Webmaster: cncbass@aol.com (webmaster <mailto:cncbass@aol.com>)

Alternative medicine: The definitive guide by the Burton Goldberg Group, Chapter: Immune support, pages 145 - 160 *The Definitive Guide* is a book that has been referred to by many as the bible of alternative health care.

List 2: Items to help with lymph drainage

Lymphatic botanicals: Medical Herbalism: A Journal for the Herbal Practitioner. Botanical Therapies for Fibrocystic Breast Disease by Jill Stansbury, N.D. Web site: http://medherb.com/92JILL.HTM Their Source: USDA Agricultural Research Service Phytochemical database. URL:http://www.ars-grin.gov/~ngrlsb/

NutraSanus, A vitabase Company: Natural Health Library: Learn about Nutritional Health, Herbal and Vitamin Supplements. Ask the Doctor: Get personalized advice directly from a Licensed Naturopathic Doctor. Products: Herbs, vitamins, minerals ect. Contact Information: Have a question about the products, policies, or procedures? Please check their Help Desk first. If you still can't find the information you need, please contact them using the information below:

Site map: http://www.nutrasanus.com/site-map.html Write: Nutrasanus.com 880-D Royal Park Drive Monroe, GA 30656 Call: 1-888-691-8134 Monday-Friday 9 am-6pm EST Email: info@nutrasanus.com <mailto:info@nutrasanus.com> We pledge a 24-hour response time (Monday through Friday) on your email requests. Please provide enough information in your email so that we can respond.

List 3: Immune stimulants

Healthnotes, Inc. HIV and AIDS Support What are the symptoms of HIV and AIDS? Contains information on medical treatments, dietary and lifestyle changes, nutritional supplements, and herbs that may be helpful. They also talk about a controversy surrounding the use of echinacea in people infected with HIV.

http://www.naturesbounty.com/vf/healthnotes/HN_live/Concern/HIV_Support.htm

Healthnotes, Inc. (HNI) is the premier provider of credible, easy-to-use health and lifestyle information. Incorporating research gathered from scientific studies published in over 550 medical and scientific journals. Founded in 1986, Healthnotes is a privately held company headquartered in Portland, Oregon USA. For more information, visit www.healthnotes.com.

United States Support and Sales

Healthnotes, Inc.

Support: 877-659-7630

Support: help@healthnotes.com

Sales: 800-659-7630

United Kingdom Support and Sales

W. Solutions

Support: 01746 766 860

Support: support@wsol.co.uk

Sales: 01746 769 888

General Contact Information

Healthnotes, Inc. Headquarters

1505 SE Gideon St., Suite 200

Portland, OR 97202

Phone: 503-234-4092

Fax: 503-234-4052

E-mail: info@healthnotes.com

Web site: http://www.healthnotes.com

List 4: Immune Modulators

"Transfer Factor Plus Advanced Formula" 4Life™

http://www.immune-system-iq.com/

Have a Question? Need Customer Service?

E-Mail: webmail.bree@gmail.com

Due to the high volume of calls we receive, you may be prompted to leave a voicemail.

609-323-7519

Please use this number if you're on an unlimited calling plan,

if you're using a cell phone, or if you're calling us from outside the U.S.

888-895-9668

Our toll free number for all other callers.

Mostly available from 9:00 AM - 6:00 PM Eastern Time, Monday - Friday.

If you have specific medical questions (e.g. dosage, which formula, etc...), please consult with your medical doctor or veterinarian. Your doctor should be aware that Transfer Factor Plus and Transfer Factor Cardio are now listed in their Physician's Desk Reference. Specific product questions can be directed to 4Life Research at 888-454-3374.

Ai/E10: Immune System Etc.com Blending science with nature. focus: immune system information. A company dedicated to helping you take control over the healing process through education and research. For more information Call Our Info Hotline bstreet books a division of Benjamin Associates Toll free (877) 454-2885 US only International calls: (586) 336-0758 email: questions@imsyssolutions.com web site: http://immunedisorders.homestead.com/supplements.html Note: their web page has changed since I quoted it. Ai/E10 is also listed in the Physician's Desk Reference for Non Prescription Drugs and Dietary Supplements.

Prime One

Much of the data for the Russian formula now used in prime one came from a web site selling the formula under the name "Soviet Secret." Unfortunately this web site is no longer available. The web addresses were http://www.coralcalciumnow.net/ Soviet-Secret.html and http://www.coralcalciumnow.net/Top-Secret-7.html

The Prime One web site however is available. The web address is http://www.amsonline.com/webpages/primeone.asp See also: http://www.iamhealthy.net/primeone.htm

Customer service 1-800-426-4267

Toll-free Order Line: 1-888-267-6733
General Questions: info@amsmainline.com
Mailing Address: 4000 N Lindsay Oklahoma City, OK 73105

AM-5000 (energy and **weight loss** solution) and Prime One are the two flagship products of AMS Health Science.

List 5: Unburdening the immune system

Colloidal Silver, Articles: Wikipedia, the free encyclopedia.

Final Note: Blood Transfusions

By transplanting a kidney along with some of the kidney donor's bone marrow, the doctors were able to cause tolerance for the kidney transplant. This is because bone marrow is part of the immune system and produces white blood cells including tolerant ones, I assume.

The thymus produces many immune cells and is part of the immune system, and as we have seen in this book, the lymph which flows through it is also part of the immune system.

Bone marrow produces blood, therefore blood is part of the immune system and if such is the case then the transfusion of blood could easily disrupt normal immune function.

Blood transfusions induce an immunosuppressive state with the recipient and that results in increased post-operative infections as well as earlier and more often re-occurrence of tumors. ~Prof. Donat R. Spahn: University of Lausanne

It has been estimated that approximately, in the United States, we can expect that 10 to 50 thousand patients a year may be dying from transfusion immuno-modulation related causes. ~Prof. Neil Blumberg: University of Rochester, New York, Director of a transfusion medicine unit and blood bank, Yr. 2002

Blood transfusions lengthen recovery time and after you've been in an accident, and both you and your immune system are weak, and you're in a hospital around a bunch of sick people, blood transfusions can be a bad idea. You could catch something.

According to the world health organization, around the globe unsafe transfusion and injection practices cause some 5,000,000 hepatitis C infections every year.

Having cancer is a bad sign as far as your immune system is concerned. If you have HIV it might be a good idea to avoid blood transfusions whenever possible.

Blood transfusions are optional. According to Prof. Roland Hetzer at least 80% of the patients would strongly favor not to have blood transfusions. ~ Yr. 2002

Today however, there are more than 100 thousand physicians and surgeons in one hundred and fifty countries who routinely treat patients without donor transfusions, according to a 28 min. video produced by the Jehovah's Witnesses entitled, "Transfusion Alternative Strategies – Simple, Safe, Effective" targeting medical professionals. The Jehovah's Witnesses are against having blood transfusions for religious reasons.

We see more than 3 thousand patients a year here that are Jehovah's witnesses and we do about two hundred and fifty to 275 major operations on them each year and what we have seen here in our population is no increased length of stay, no increased mortality, and in fact it seems to be somewhat decreased. ~Prof. Stephen M. Cohn, University of Miami, Florida, Yr. 2002

We are only just beginning to understand the immune system. It's amazing, just how much we don't know.

If you would like more information on this topic you can look it up on the internet. Subjects that you might want to include would be:

- Blood transfusions and the immune system, or as described by Prof. Spahn: an Immunosuppressive state
- Blood transfusion alternatives
- Blood fractions
- A medical directive incase you get in an accident

For a really bad accident you might want to reconsider but a great majority of blood transfusions are given out just as a matter of procedure and not because anyone really needs them. Most often saline solution would work just as well.

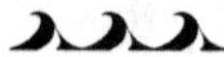

Finally

Good luck with your diseases, or whatever else you have. If you ever want to hear my words again or if you just want to remember what you've read, you can read the map-summery which is located at the back of this book. It's been reworded and you might learn just a few things you didn't know before. Our story's not over yet as the ending lies with you. Good luck tomorrow and see you later my friend.

Jason Mc Kenna

Map of Book

In the map summery you can scan for a particular part of the book you want to read. It is also excellent for review. You may find things you missed before since it's been reworded.

Introduction

The first part of this book is about a theory which explains the secret of cancer and AIDS's invincibility to the immune system. In order to understand the latest options for treatment though, which were derived from this theory, you would have to read about the theory first.
The Theory

Slow Viruses

HIV belongs to a subgroup of retroviruses known as lentiviruses, or "slow" viruses. A number of slow virus infections have in fact been caused by conventional viruses. For instance, a case of Measles can turn into a slow viral infection.

Early Events in HIV Infection

At first, HIV replicates rapidly, seeding various organs as it travels through the bloodstream, particularly the **lymphoid organs.** Two to 4 weeks after exposure to HIV, up to 70 percent of HIV-infected people suffer flu-like symptoms. Their immune systems fight back with **killer T cells** and **antibodies**, dramatically reducing HIV levels. So, the immune system could easily win if only it continued to attack HIV as it did to begin with. A person may then remain free of HIV-related symptoms for years, despite continuous replication of HIV in the lymphoid organs which were seeded during the acute phase of infection. Perhaps somehow the virus tampered with part of the immune system causing it to recognize the virus as a self antigen, or part of the body. This would account for the lack of symptoms.

Early in the course of HIV infection, people may lose HIV-specific CD4+ T cell responses. Also, certain subsets of killer T cells that recognize HIV may become depleted or dysfunctional. Like cancer, for whatever reason the immune system no longer attacks HIV as it should.

Cancer does not cause any symptoms because the immune system does not respond to it. The flu-like symptoms of HIV are caused by the immune system responding to the virus and not the virus itself. If those symptoms are absent, that means the immune responses that cause them are absent. The fact that normal viruses can cause slow viral infections shows that a slow infection is more of a condition that can be triggered than just an infection.

Vaccines do not always work against slow viruses due to the onset of immunological tolerance soon after infection. To cure AIDS permanently you would have to figure out how the virus triggers tolerance and stop it. You will know if your cure works when the patient starts showing symptoms. An AIDS patient will start showing flu-like symptoms and an SSEP patient will come down with the measles.

Part 2

There are 2 main types of tolerance, B cells and T cells. HIV infects T cells so we'll look there first. In the thymus, antigen presenting cells present self antigens to T cells so they'll see self antigens as part of the human body and not attack them. Perhaps the antigen presenting cells are presenting viral antigens along with self antigens.

Lack of Co-stimulation

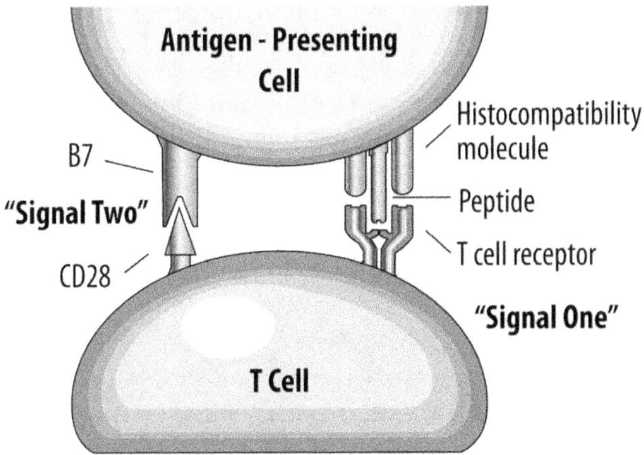

This is called co-stimulation, which is needed to activate T cells. If the T cell fails to receive "signal two," it dies by apoptosis.

The binding of a T cell's antigen receptors to an antigen is not enough to cause the T cell to carry out an immune reaction against it. For that, the T cell would also have to receive a **second signal** from the cell presenting the antigen (the APC). The cells presenting the body's own self antigens fail to provide signal two and this causes tolerance to the antigens they present so that our immune systems won't attack our own bodies. Once HIV infects a person there may be so many viral antigens in the lymphoid system that some APCs might pick them up instead of self antigens. They would then present HIV antigens to T Cells as if they were the body's own antigens, causing tolerance to them.

Part 3

All slow virus infections start off with a long latent period before symptoms (the immune response) appear. During this time the virus builds up its antigens in order to cause tolerance. The more antigens there are, the more they get mixed up with self antigens. A person may remain free of HIV-related symptoms for years despite viral replication. For a long time there is only a small amount of tolerance so for a while it's not so bad.

Suppressor T cells

It is now clear that if T cells are not co-stimulated they act as potent suppressor cells, suppressing the immune response.

Viral antigens could bind directly to T cells without APCs to provide co-stimulation or, more likely, antigen presenting cells could have presented HIV or cancer antigens as self antigens. This would produce suppressor T cells which would shelter some of the viruses. Over time the number of viruses would increase little by little with increasing tolerance.

Elephantiasis

It's caused by a worm that makes nests in person's lymph system. Infection can linger for years or decades. Carcinoma**:** It spreads to other parts of the body mainly through the lymph vessels.

All this happens around the immune system, so suppressor cells could work by breaking the chain of signals that stimulates an immune response. If such is the case, it might be necessary to kill those suppressor T cells

Suppressor T cells may be involved in how animals tolerate pregnancy without rejecting the fetus, tolerance for kidney transplants and even self tolerance so we might not want to get rid of them after all.

Once an antigen is absent so is the stimuli for an immune response. Theoretically, that's why the symptoms disappear after we're not sick anymore. I wonder if suppressor cells could work by blocking the stimuli for the immune response.

They say, HIV disrupts signaling molecules that normally regulate a person's immune response. That's an awfully complex task for a virus to do. In cell cultures CD4+ T cells could be turned off by activation signals from HIV. In reality though, the T cells were probably turned off by APCs presenting HIV antigens without co-stimulation, or... the activation signals could have just come from the suppressor T cells that were produced.

Suppressor T cells are important in self-tolerance which prevents autoimmune diseases. Suppressor T cells may also be involved in self-cancer-tolerance.

Induced tolerance is tolerance to external antigens which prevents allergic reactions. HIV is like an external antigen (such as pollen) and can induce tolerance as well. Allergens and tuberculosis enter our lungs and both may induce tolerance.

Supporting Evidence

Vaccines: and the "window of immunogenicity."

Too much or too little antigen may induce tolerance rather than an active immune response.

The ratio of helper T cells to suppressor T cells

AIDS is characterized by a very low ratio of helper T cells to suppressor T cells.

According to the encyclopedia, Wikipedia,

Some pathogens may have evolved to manipulate regulatory T cells to suppress the host. For example, regulatory T cell activity is reported to increase in retroviral infections. HIV is a retrovirus.

HIV actually stands for Human Immunodeficiency Virus.

The Solution

We could either remove the viral antigens so they can't cause tolerance anymore, or we could undo the tolerance they have created. To undo the tolerance would cause our immune systems to attack our own bodies.

If the problem is that antigens could bind directly to un-primed T cell without APC co-stimulation then if we had more antigen presenting cells, less antigens would bind to T cells on their own. People who get cancer probably suffer from a lack of "antigen presenting cells" (APCs).

But wouldn't that be more like a rare genetic condition? And what about carcinogens? If APCs cause the self presentation of foreign antigens, this idea of a lack is unfounded. Increasing their numbers could even make things worse, although that is unknown.

Another Theory

Preventing APCs from presenting HIV as a self antigen could correct the tolerance.

Polysaccharides cause APCs to present HIV as foreign more often. They do this by being foreign substances in the body, stimulating the immune system. The more often HIV is seen as foreign the less often it is seen as a self antigen.

This only makes APCs mistake HIV for self antigens less often, but it would still help. The real benefit here comes from the small immune response it would initiate. This could wipe out some of the viral antigens and thereby lessen the tolerance. So, it turns out, we can lessen the antigens, but to do this we must first study the lymph system.

Lymph System:

Lymph carries nutrients from the blood to the cells and carries wastes away from them. It also acts as a mini sewer system removing wastes and toxins from the body. During the flu, the nodes at the neck may visibly swell with collected waste products. Lymph should be clear but it can also become milk-like to yogurt to cottage cheese. Thick, gel-like lymph fluid will not flow as it should and can congest the lymph system. The nodes filter lymph fluid but if blocked, they also become storage points for waste (and antigens).

Conclusions

When HIV antigens build up, APCs can't help but pick them up instead of self antigens. People who are prone to cancer probably suffer from poor lymph circulation. This would cause cancer antigens to build up to levels approaching that of self antigens.

Suppressor T cells get created immediately around the tumor due to its antigens. Cancer may only be able to spread to where its antigens (and tolerance) have spread first. Any cancer cells that move out of this tolerant area get destroyed. You don't often see a tumor with a lot of surface area. They're bulbous. Even HIV has a tendency to build up in little clusters in lymph nodes, just like a tumor. Any cancer cells or

HIV that moves out of this tolerant area get destroyed more easily.

The degradation of the immune system

If the flu can make the nodes swell at the neck, just think of what AIDS can do. Large amounts of the virus become trapped in networks of follicular dendritic cells. This leads to the breakdown of the lymph node architecture replacing it with scar tissue. That takes a lot of antigens and that is exactly the problem. Clearing the antigens is vital and absolutely necessary

What can be done to clear the lymph system?

To keep it clear, stay healthy and take care of yourself. Sounds weak, read it anyway.

Stress depresses your immune system and wears you out. You need to recuperate.

Exercise moves the lymph fluid and can increase lymphatic flow up to threefold.

Deep breathing drains lymph fluid into the thoracic duct. It causes lymph to flow.

Diet: Wheat and dairy clogs the lymph system.

Stomach: Digest your food or it will putrefy in your intestine which produces acid. The acid will then penetrate your intestinal wall and lower the pH of your entire body.

Constipation: When the intestinal walls are impacted the lymph fluid can't drain into your intestines. Wastes get backed up into your abdominal tissues & your lymph nodes bloat with wastes.

Water Your bladder and kidneys are also important for eliminating waste. Water will flush you out and keep your insides clean. Not drinking enough means you're not peeing enough and your body gets polluted.

Liver The liver filters out toxins, poison and viruses from your blood. The liver dumps many of its toxins into the bile and then into the intestines. The coffee enema is a popular liver cleanser. It opens the bile ducts causing bile to flow. The liver can then dump many of its toxins into the bile and get rid of them within minutes.

Spleen The spleen is similar to the lymph nodes, except it filters blood instead of lymph.

Celery seed has been used to treat certain diseases of the liver and spleen. It is also used to clean out the body of its excess water and wastes, especially uric acid.

A Bad Habit

The story of Nila, a lot of soda pop, and the dangers of quitting a bad habit too quickly. I'm sure you remember it. The moral: don't shock your body with a sudden change, even a healthy one.

The Lymph fluid

Manual lymphatic drainage (MLD) is an important massage treatment in lymphedema. It is designed to move the excess fluid away from swollen areas so it can drain away.

Vibratory machines (The "Lymphstar Pro") A simple vibratory device might be best for you. You've got to keep your fluids moving. The primary channels for release of lymph are in the crease of the groin and armpits. If they get clogged, this could be why breast and prostate cancer are some of the most common cancers.

Flexitouch® System A garment with chambers that inflate and deflate to help move your lymph fluid along.

Infrared heat lamp Such a lamp can increase the circulation around tumors and reduce swollen lymph nodes.

Alzheimer's: The brain is steeped in its own proteins which build up to the point of forming plaques. Such a lamp could increase the circulation of cerebrospinal fluid (in you back) and make your brain cleaner. Point lamp at back, don't bake your brain.

You're going to need more than proper diet and exercise to cure AIDS.

First the fine print: You must unclog the lymph system. Herbs could help with this.

Fine print on Immunostimulants: If it's not prescription it should be fairly safe. A popular theory is that the immune system of an AIDS patent is already over-stimulated from the AIDS virus so you'd think that you would not want to stimulate the immune system any further, but there is a new theory that the AIDS virus actually suppresses the immune system. If so, the immune system would not actually be over-stimulated and under these circumstances you would not have to worry about over-stimulation or immune stimulants.

List 1:
Agents for boosting the activity of antigen presenting cells

Mushrooms

beta-glucan A type of polysaccharide studied as a treatment for cancer.

lentinan A type of beta-glucan. It has been studied in Japan as a treatment for cancer.

Coriolus Mushroom: Commonly known as the "**turkey tail**" in North America, boosts **antigen-presenting cell** function of macrophages, thus overall immune function.

The reishi mushroom: Has anti-tumor activities and modulates many components of the immune system.

List 2:
Items to help with lymph drainage

Maitake mushroom, researched for its ability to prevent or treat cancer and as a treatment for HIV infection, Maitake mushroom contains polysaccharides so it would also fit into list number one.

Lymphagogue: An agent which makes lymph more watery so it flows more easily.

Lymphatic botanicals: Herbs that can assist the lymphatic system in clearing congestion and wastes. Lymph movers include: pokeweed, blue flag, New Jersey tea, and cleavers (bedstraw).

Cayenne peppers were used to reduce swollen lymph glands caused by tuberculosis. **Prickly ash bark**, **Stillingia root**, and **wild indigo root** are all used to treat lymph fluid. **Celery seed** extract is a diuretic and it can also be used to clean out the body. **Asparagus tea** and **water pills** are also diuretics.

List 3: Immune Stimulants

Immunostimulants may help to counter-act suppression, since they have the opposite effect

Herbs

Cat's Claw, Inner Bark (Uncaria tomentosa) stimulates the activity of T cells.

Astragalus Root (Astragalus membranaceus) The body can develop a tolerance to an adaptogenic herb if taken for too long at a time.

Echinacea Root (Echinacea purpurea)

Cautions A controversy has surrounded the use of echinacea in people infected with HIV.

SO WHY DO PEOPLE WITH HIV USE ECHINACEA?

Because it stimulates the immune system, and for colds or the flu. Some believe it is a bad idea to stimulate an immune system that is already overactive. Yet there is absolutely no experimental evidence to indicate any dangers whatsoever.

Some doctors believe the immune system is already being over stimulated. Yet the whole premise of this book is that the immune system is actually being suppressed. If true then there would be no danger of over-stimulating the immune system.

Experimental evidence suggests echinacea could actually help people with HIV. One double-blind trial found echinacea greatly increased immune activity against HIV.

Bee stings as immune stimulants

Bee and scorpion stings are also immune stimulants. One doctor just south of where I live intentionally has his patients get stung by bees for their arthritis. You may want to buy your own pet emperor scorpion. You only need to get stung once a week or so, so it's not too bad.

Tarantulas

A tarantula bite "may" be less painful than the sting of a bee, depending on the species, but they may also have irritating hairs or large fangs that can leave little puncture marks.

Allergic to be stings

A simple cure would be to just go out and get stung on a routine basis. Eat an eighth of a peanut a day, if you are mildly allergic to peanuts. Eventually you should become much more tolerant of what you are allergic to.

Mild arthritis

Theoretically, the maximum dosage of echinacea could act like a bee sting. Antihistamine only seems to act as a potent anti-inflammatory for arthritis when used with a diuretic. The diuretic removes uric acid crystals that would otherwise trigger an immune response and the antihistamine keeps what's left of the immune response under control.

This two part treatment is a bit of a parallel to the treatment discussed in this book. Lymphagogues and diuretics remove excess antigens that would otherwise suppress an immune response and immune stimulants cause the immune system to react.

Aspirin may reduce joint pain and arthritic swelling around joints making the joints last longer. An anti-inflammatory may also be useful for chronically inflamed lymph nodes like in AIDS.

Celery seed is especially effective against gout and gout induced arthritis. In gout, uric acid crystals build up in the joints, especially where circulation is sluggish. The cold can also decrees circulation by causing blood vesicles to constrict. Cayenne pepper powder put into capsules can be used to increase circulation.

Celery seed is a diuretic and can be used in getting rid of the uric acid crystals in the joints. Diuretics may be more effective for getting rid of some things than lymph thinners are.

Stimulants - Tree Extracts, Herbs, Flowers, Mushrooms and Such

These stimulants push parts of the immune system to work faster. Together, they can be quite effective for a short while.

Immune System Stimulation Has a Limited Effect

Excessive stimulation, like stress, can take a toll on the immune system and wear it down.

Drugs

There are a number of prescription drugs, but for that you'd have to ask your doctor.

List 4: Immune Modulators

Immune modulators increase or decrease the activity of each element of the Immune System as needed. They bring an underactive immune system up and an overactive immune system down; excellent for those with out of whack immune systems.

Chronic fatigue syndrome: found to have both high and low ratios of helper T cells. This could be a sign of a poorly regulated immune system however... Chronic fatigue has many things in common with HIV and slow viral infections. It is also called Post-Viral Fatigue Syndrome and immune suppression may be involved. If so, the same treatments for cancer and HIV could be used against chronic fatigue. However, immune modulators would not be enough by themselves.

Transfer Factor Plus Advanced Formula

Independent lab tests prove it increases the Natural Killer (NK) cell activity by 437%. This NK function is what destroys (lyses) virus-infected cells and tumor cells. Echinacea only increased this function by 43%. You'll remember it increases TNF-alpha. NK cell activity in chronic fatigue, cancer, and chronic viral infections is usually low so this might help 437%.

Ai/E10

Ai/E10 can help bring under- or overactive immune systems

into balance. It restores communication pathways, regulates and strengthens immune function. Communication pathways are important when it comes to suppressor T cells.

Thymus Extracts

Thymus extracts have been shown to normalize the ratio of T helper cells to suppressor cells, whether the ratio is low (as in AIDS and cancer) or high (as in allergies or arthritis).

Adaptogens

Adaptogens are often combined. This is more effective than either plant used alone.

Astragalus *(Astragalus membranaceus)*

Actions: Immune stimulant; adaptogenic. **Uses:** Tonic and endurance remedy. Not an acute remedy, like echinacea, but for long-term use to improve immune function. This herb is able to foster normal immune response in cancer and AIDS patients. Astragalus has many potential applications and it has no known harmful side effects.

Supreme Protector

It is composed of the three kings of defense: Reishi, Astragalus and **Cordyceps.**

Protector 2000

It contains the three strongest immune modulators known to Chinese herbalism. Agaricus mushroom, reishi Mushroom, and lycium polysaccharides.

Prime One -

Stress and not getting enough rest could very well be degrading your health. Adaptogens help your body to build itself up. They cause the body to respond to stress as though it were exercise. Too many immune stimulants can stress the immune system, but now all that stress could be converted into exercise. Stimulants could even be used to exercise the immune system and build it up, theoretically. A suppressed immune system probably wouldn't get much exercise without them. You must give your immune system something to adapt to for adaptogens to work.

The Russians secretly developed a formula to give them an edge over everyone else. The formula is now considered the number one stress relief product in the world. It is a formula of seven adaptogens. Once given to KGB agents and Olympic teams, this same formula is now used in "Prime One."

Supercharges Immunity Adaptogens are powerful immune modulators. Prime One also gives you more energy. If you are more active, then you can be more proactive in taking care of yourself. Coffee will also give you more energy, but it works by allowing you to overexert yourself. Avoided long term use of stimulants. Only use what makes you stronger.

List 5:
Unburdening the immune system

We all have germs, but an AIDS patient can be like an old tree just covered in fungus. This can put quite a burden on your immune system (or lymph system). There are only mild symptoms with this so there may be some tolerance to the bacteria. An AIDS patient could form tolerance to bacteria easily with their clogged lymph fluid. If the immune system is just extremely tolerant then the immune system hasn't really been destroyed! It just looks like it so it's not really too late. In order to help the immune system to recuperate, get rid of all the secondary infections.

Goldenseal

Used as an all-around disinfectant, believed to only effect in the gastrointestinal track. Main use: Colds and flu, upper respiratory infections, and chronic fatigue syndrome.

Colloidal silver

It is a non-toxic anti-microbial, viricide, bactericide, fungicide and disinfectant. It will not hurt friendly bacteria in the digestive tract and other areas of the body. It was once used by physicians as a mainstream antibiotic till sulfa drugs and penicillin appeared.

Colloidal silver spry sprayed on Hong Kong subways as a public health measure. Silver is now used to sterilize recycled water aboard the Mir Space Station.

Considerations

Colloidal Silver is non-toxic, but it could kill a lot of bad bacteria. You'll then have to remove the dead germs from your body and lymph. Drink plenty of fluid. One man drank 16 ounces of colloidal silver a day for four days in a row. He felt fine! If you decide to make your own colloidal silver at home, instructions are on the internet. You might want a little more than a tinny bottle from the store for an advanced illness. Silver nitrate could turn your skin blue and sterling silver contains copper. Don't drink copper.

Colloidal silver spray

If you have tuberculosis you could spray colloidal silver into your lungs as you inhale. As it turns out, they already make spray bottles of colloidal silver just for this purpose.

HIV does not have a 100% mortality rate, so don't give up hope. Believe in yourself. The progression of a disease is not up to the germ. It's up to your immune system.

A Simple Basic Test Run [Just to try it out]

This probably won't cure you. It's just to see if it could help you to recover or not. Then you could decide if you want to pursue the matter further. For the most affordable remedy I can think of, try:

"Red Clover Stillingia" from "Herb Pharm"

"A Diuretic" Celery seed

"Colloidal Silver" from "Source Naturals"

"All Thymus" from "Natural Sources"

"Reishi mushroom" or other mushrooms

"Echinacea and Astragalus"

Refined Test run:

1. Lymph thinner / Stillingia
2. Diuretic / celery seed
3. Immune stimulant / Echinacea
4. Adaptogen / Astragalus
5. Pacing / exercise

The Real Treatment

You might want to specialize in stimulants, adaptogens, lymph thinners, and a diuretic. Counteracting tolerance and removing excessive antigens is at the heart of this treatment. However, the real treatment (not the test run) is mildly expensive and you have to take a lot of things.

Antibiotics are not part of the real treatment as they do not directly bring down the level of tolerance or affect the immune system. You can either take a little echinacea long term, or take a lot of it with breaks in between. Taking a lot with breaks is recommended. You must take exercise with this treatment. Thinning the lymph won't do any good if it's not moving and pacing is currently the most effective single treatment for chronic fatigue syndrome.

What Comes First?

If you have HIV, you could take echinacea with scorpion stings during your breaks. The key to this treatment is to take everything you can and as much as possible; (1st) stimulants (2d) lymph thinners (3d) diuretics (4th) adaptogens (5th) modulators. If you don't plan on getting stung often, then lymph thinners and diuretics take first place.

Gauging Effectiveness

If you have HIV and then get flu-like symptoms; that might just be an immune response.

What to Use

All of the ingredients mentioned in the test run could easily be replaced by others. Want to kick it up a notch? A much more effective and expensive treatment would be: Miracle mineral solution (sodium chlorite), Transfer Factor Plus, Prime One, cleavers or New Jersey tea; plus diuretic and exercise.

What you can do to help yourself

Whatever treatment you need, it does not have to be an act of self mutilation. Exercise can be light just as long as it's consistent. The main reason why so many diets fail is because diets only work while you're on them.

You can't put forth much effort without motivation.

You need to daydream about making things a whole lot better. Then you'll have a desire. Was anyone on earth really qualified to tackle cancer and AIDS? I was not but I did. You may have to make decisions in your treatment even if you are not qualified to do so. You could also help your friends and neighbors if they have cancer or HIV. It is possible to use my method without prescription drugs, so it should be quite safe. It should also be much easier on the patient than whatever they are going through now. Here are some various things you might want to look up on the internet:

- Co-stimulation & antigen presenting cells
- Suppressor T cells, also known as Regulatory T Cells
- (Immuno-regulatory agents) such as drugs and herbs
- How to drain the lymph system of toxins. ~This is the most important thing

Don't stop reading now because this book isn't over yet, as the ending lies with you.

Author Jason Mc Kenna

Sources: Organized by book chapter

The Theory

The Solution

List 2: Items to help with lymph drainage

List 3: Immune stimulants

List 4: Immune Modulators

List 5: Unburdening the immune system

Colloidal Silver, Articles: Wikipedia, the free encyclopedia.

Final Note: Blood Transfusions

By transplanting a kidney along with some of the kidney donor's bone marrow, the doctors were able to cause tolerance for the kidney transplant. Scientists have shown that bone marrow can be involved in some kinds of tolerance. This is because bone marrow produces white blood cells including tolerant ones, I think. The thymus produces many immune cells, and as we have seen in this book, the lymph fluid which flows through it is also part of the immune system.

Bone marrow produces blood, therefore blood is part of the immune system. If so, then the transfusion of blood could easily disrupt normal immune function. Blood transfusions induce an immunosuppressive state with the recipient. This results in more frequent post-operative infections and re-occurrence of tumors. Thousands of patients may be dying of transfusion immuno-modulation related causes. If you already have cancer, blood transfusions should be avoided whenever possible. Blood transfusions are optional. Thousands of physicians routinely treat patients without donor transfusions.

We are only just beginning to understand the immune system. It's amazing, just how much we don't know. If you would like more information on this topic you can look it up on the internet. Subjects that you might want to include would be:

- Blood transfusions and the immune system, or an Immunosuppressive state
- Blood transfusion alternatives
- Blood fractions
- A medical directive incase you get in an accident

For a really bad accident you might want to reconsider, but most blood transfusions are given out just as a matter of procedure. Most often saline solution would work just as well.

Finally

Good luck with your problems. If you ever want to hear my words again you can always re-read this book. With what you know now, you may see it in a new light. Our story's not over yet as the ending lies with you. Good luck and I'll be here if you need me.

Jason Mc Kenna

www.ingramcontent.com/pod-product-compliance
Lightning Source LLC
Chambersburg PA
CBHW051542170526
45165CB00002B/846

* 9 7 8 1 4 3 2 7 3 9 7 7 5 *